Patient Communication for First Responders and EMS Personnel

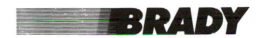

Patient Communication for First Responders and EMS Personnel:
The First Hour of Trauma

Donald Trent Jacobs

Brady
A Prentice Hall Division
Englewood Cliffs, New Jersey 07632

Library of Congress Cataloging-in-Publication Data

Jacobs, Donald T.
    Patient communication for first responders and EMS personnel : the
first hour of trauma / Donald Trent Jacobs.
      p. cm.
    Includes bibliographical references.
    Includes index.
    ISBN 0-89303-732-X

    1. Emergency medical technician and patient. 2. Communication in
emergency medicine. I. Title
    [DNLM: 1. Communication. 2. Emergency Medical Services.
  3. Professional-Patient Relations.   WX 215 J16p]
  RC86.3.J33 1991
  362.1′8—dc20
  DNLM/DLC
  for Library of Congress   90-15110
                                                        CIP

Editorial/production supervision and
   interior design: Wordcrafters Editorial Services, Inc.
Cover design: Karen Stephens
Cover photo: FPG International © Peterson, Bob 1989
Manufacturing buyer: Mary McCartney and Ed O'Dougherty

This book can be made available to business and organizations at a
special discount when ordered in large quantities. For more information
contact: Prentice-Hall, Inc., Special Sales and Markets, College Division,
Englewood Cliffs, N.J. 07632.

© 1991 by Prentice-Hall, Inc.
A Division of Simon & Schuster
Englewood Cliffs, New Jersey 07632

Printed in the United States of America
10 9 8 7 6 5 4 3 2 1

ISBN 0-89303-732-X

Prentice-Hall International (UK) Limited, *London*
Prentice-Hall of Australia Pty. Limited, *Sydney*
Prentice-Hall Canada Inc., *Toronto*
Prentice-Hall Hispanoamericana, S.A., *Mexico*
Prentice-Hall of India Private Limited, *New Delhi*
Prentice-Hall of Japan Inc., *Tokyo*
Simon & Schuster Asia Pte. Ltd., *Singapore*
Editora Prentice-Hall do Brasil, Ltda., *Rio de Janeiro*

This textbook is dedicated to those who stand ready to apply their utmost resources toward the rescue of another life.

About the Author

Dr. Jacobs earned his doctorate in Health Psychology while working as a fire fighter and emergency medical technician (EMT). After earning his degree, he continued as a professional prehospital care provider for almost a decade before beginning a private hypnotherapy practice in Novato, California. During this time he field-tested the approaches to patient communication presented in this text.

Dr. Jacobs has also personally experimented with the techniques relating to the mind-body connection. He has walked on fire, undergone abdominal surgery without anesthesia, survived remote wilderness catastrophes, and has calmed wild horses.

Dr. Jacobs is the author of seven other books, including a book on physical fitness and stress management for fire fighters. He currently resides on a ranch in northern California with his wife and daughter.

Contents

Foreword

I have known Donald Jacobs for many years and am delighted that he has put together in very readable form the summation of his experience with burned, hemorrhaging, traumatized, and frightened people.

His knowledge about the semantics of communication with conscious and unconscious people in crises comes from firsthand experience on the scene and careful research into the behavior characteristics of frightened people in altered states of consciousness.

He has observed the remarkable resources available to traumatized people when their medical attendants know how to activate these resources. He has seen wounded people stop hemorrhaging, turn off pain, and accelerate their healing potential in response to words that are honestly and caringly offered by those who are first on the scene.

All of us need to study the messages contained here and to practice with Dr. Jacobs's art. Any of us may, at any moment, be confronted with catastrophic life situations where the knowledge we have absorbed here may save lives. As he points out in his final chapter, our planet is facing grave dangers from the careless actions of its human inhabitants. We must think, act, and speak appropriately *now*. This book is timely in a world of catastrophic events. It should be in every person's library and should be studied carefully by all of us.

DAVID B. CHEEK, M.D., FACS, FACOG
Santa Barbara, California
September 28, 1989

Preface

Most texts on emergency medical care briefly mention the importance of calming and reassuring the patient and of using proper words and manner of speech when rendering first aid. For example, in *Emergency Care and Transportation of the Sick and Injured* by the American Academy of Orthopaedic Surgeons, the authors state the following:

> This means being extremely careful about what is said at the scene. During periods of great stress, words that seem immaterial or are uttered in jest might become fixed in the patient's mind and cause untold harm. Conversation at the scene must be appropriate.

But what *is* "appropriate" conversation? Why do words have such power? What potential is there for the *positive* influence of words? How can we learn to project calmness and reassurance in the face of frightening events and life-threatening injuries or illness? In short, what is the most effective way to communicate with a person in trauma?

Patient Communication for First Responders and EMS Personnel: The First Hour of Trauma answers these questions and presents communication strategies that can tap the inner resources of a patient. It is based on research that continues to show that certain kinds of verbal and nonverbal communication with people in stress can influence virtually every nervous system function and its result—from bleeding and blood pressure to inflammation and immune response. It is also based on evidence indicating that proper communication can increase the effectiveness of standard medical treatment.

This book presents guidelines, strategies, and techniques that can be used in the field, not only to prevent "untold harm," but also to enhance a patient's natural survival and healing capabilities. It is targeted for professional and volunteer medical emergency personnel, but it can easily be used by anyone who might find themselves attending a sick, injured, or frightened person. With this audience in mind, the terms *first responder, rescuer, first-aider, EMT, paramedic,* and so on, will be used throughout the text and should be considered interchangeable. (Professional dispatchers who must speak with frightened reporting parties on the telephone will also benefit from this book.)

Patient Communication for First Responders and EMS Personnel: The First Hour of Trauma might be described as a first aid book that is more concerned with the perceptions of the patient than with those of the rescuer. It thus expands the boundaries of primary care so that anyone can learn to take immediate advantage of the mind-body connection that is rapidly becoming the focus of interest in science and medicine.

Research tells us that, to the extent our thoughts, beliefs, and attitudes are negative, we send messages to every part of our body that discourage optimal functioning. To the extent that they are positive, we send messages that encourage survival and health. When we are frightened, confused, or seriously injured or ill, our thoughts are often dependent on what is told to us by confident voices. When these voices know how to direct positive responses, they can be life saving, especially when the communication occurs within the first hour post trauma, before stressful reactions become more deeply rooted.*

---

*When negative emotions and inappropriate interpretations become deeply rooted in a medical emergency patient, they can remain self-defeating for many years, even after physical recovery. Many posttrauma stress disorders have been traced back to less than optimal communication at the emergency scene. Thus, proper communication cannot only enhance recovery immediately after trauma, it can also prevent future anxiety syndromes. This is especially true for young people.

This text will help you become that confident, knowing voice. Note: It is important to be aware that the communication strategies described in this book are an adjunct to standard emergency medical care. They will not replace and should not interrupt such care.

Acknowledgments

My sincere appreciation to the following people.

To the paramedics and fire fighters who first tolerated, then supported, my work in the field, including Frank Neer, David Carr, and Jack McBurt.

To the physicians and psychologists who broke tradition and inspired me to share this information with first responders, including David Cheek, M.D.; Rashiha Jama, Ph.D.; Dabney Ewin, M.D.; Gerald Kaplan, M.D.; Lee Balance, M.D.; Tom Stern, M.D.; Helmet Relinger, M.D.; Jessie Miller, Ph.D.; Thomas Elmendorf, M.D.; Larry Moore, Ph.D.; M. Erik Wright, M.D., Ph.D.; and Beatrice Wright, Ph.D.

To the many pioneering researchers whose work encouraged me to see the value of the mind-body connection in the emergency field, especially to David Cheek, M.D.; Dabney Ewin, M.D.; M. Erik

Wright, M.D., Ph.D; Irving Oyle, M.D.; Gil Boyne; and Norman Cousins.

To the editors who published my articles on this subject; to Claire Merrick, whose belief made this book possible; and to Kate Templeton, who dared to edit my rough draft and type the final manuscript.

And, finally, to my wife Beatrice, whose confidence in me has nurtured my own positive images.

Epigraph

This material presents both an opportunity and a challenge to all prehospital care personnel. The opportunity is to develop patient communication at a level previously unknown, a level that may enhance positive and possibly lifesaving physiological responses.

The challenge is to break through the barriers of bias, preconception, and mind-set that deter objective evaluation.

THOMAS ELMENDORF, M.D.

Past President
California Medical Association

Introduction

ORIENTATION

When you communicate with a person in trauma, your words touch the tip of an iceberg. Beneath the surface numerous associations and responses can be set in motion. Often these occur at the unconscious (subconscious) level. When they do, every word, phrase, sentence, pause, voice inflection and gesture can initiate automatic psycho-physiologic effects.

As was mentioned in the preface, this sensitive receptivity to words and gestures is most acute during the first hour post trauma. If after this amount of time external communication is not received, people in trauma begin to rely on their own internal communication. Using past experience or learned associations, patients begin to interpret their predicament and respond to it accordingly. During the first hour or so, however, it appears that injured, frightened or confused people focus their entire attention on trying to understand the situation by waiting for appropriate directions. This may be why people tend to freeze during surprising or sudden emergencies until someone finally shouts, "Don't just stand there, call a doctor!"

Unfortunately, the past associations of most people are not optimal for coping with medical emergencies. Instead, they create added stress. It is generally agreed that mental stress contributes significantly to the majority of medical problems. Medical emergencies are no exception. Stress impairs the immune system and weakens organs and glands.* When combined with physical injury, it impedes recovery.

The art of effective communication with persons in trauma thus relates to using words and gestures to minimize negative stress and maximize healing processes that can occur at multiple levels of consciousness. This requires speaking the language of the unconscious mind as well as that of the conscious or analytical mind.

It is the working assumption of this text that the language of the unconscious mind pertains to the concept of "imagery." Beneath the tip of the iceberg that represents our simple, objective language, words trigger associations that form images within the mind. Research shows that such images can direct nervous system functions that are usually considered involuntary.

Imagery, in this context, is not necessarily defined as vivid pictures in the mind's eye. Rather, imagery describes those internal perceptions that may involve all of our senses. Like dreams, images can be simple and clear, or they can be complicated and vague. In either case, the chapters that follow are intended to help you understand and utilize those communication strategies that evoke possible life saving images in the patient. To help you remember the fundamental aspects of such strategies, the mnemonic C R E D I B L E (representing the words Confidence, Rapport, Expectation, Directives, Images, Believability, Literalness, and Enthusiasm) is presented. The chapters of the book follow the guidelines represented by this mnemonic.

Part I teaches ways to increase the believability of what you say to the patient. Chapter 1 offers information that illustrates the effectiveness of this kind of communication. Chapter 2 teaches you how to project Confidence at the emergency scene. Chapter 3 shows you how to gain and maintain proper Rapport with the person in trauma.

---

*The biological stress response was designed to prevent injury by mobilizing fight or flight capabilities. For example, immune and digestive systems are shut down. Blood pressure is increased. After the injury, when the danger of further trauma is passed, this response is no longer helpful. Psychological concerns, however, are nonetheless interpretted by the nervous system as another physical threat requiring fight or flight.

Chapter 4 describes how to build the patient's Expectations for a positive, hopeful future.

Part II offers guidelines for giving the emergency patient Directives that can tap his or her own powerful coping abilities. Chapter 5 begins teaching specific guidelines for such communication. Chapters 6 through 9 use the C R E D I B L E mnemonic's suffix (Images, Believability, Literalness, and Enthusiasm) to present basic rules and illustrations that will help assure that directives to the patient will be successful. Chapters 10 through 17 discuss particular emergency situations and offer phrasing examples that use the techniques described in earlier chapters. (The examples are based on actual case studies where they were used effectively. It is suggested that they be memorized, then modified to suit unique situations and communication styles.) Chapter 18 gives information on the use of *self talk* and belief systems that can help you survive a personal trauma. Finally, Chapter 19 tells how the same principles of language and thoughts that can dramatically influence human biology can contribute to the saving of the planet.

LEGAL AND ETHICAL CONSIDERATIONS

Consider this hypothetical situation. Two paramedics respond to an emergency call for help. When they arrive on the scene they find a thirty-two-year-old female complaining of nausea and acute back pain. She states that she has been passing blood in her urine for several hours. The paramedics follow standard care protocols and proceed to transport the patient to the hospital in the ambulance. Riding in the back of the ambulance with the patient along with one of the paramedics is the woman's five-year-old daughter.

On the way to the hospital, the patient's vital signs begin to diminish. Seriously concerned and emotionally distraught by the tears of the little girl, the paramedic in the back says to the paramedic who is driving, "Hurry up John, she won't make it if we don't get there soon."

The woman is dead on arrival and CPR efforts are unsuccessful. Shortly after, the woman's husband learns from his daughter that one of the paramedics said, "she won't make it." He sues the county the paramedics work for, claiming that the paramedic's words were responsible for his wife giving up hope.

Is the county or the paramedic liable for negligence? Of course, we can only guess what the verdict would be. There is, however, a real possibility that the paramedic's words may have had an influence on the patient's survival. As mentioned earlier, the Academy of

Orthopaedic Surgeons talks about words causing "untold harm." Grant and Murray also state in their textbook on *Emergency Care* that "the manner in which the EMT cares for his patient may in some respects be as important as the emergency care measures themselves. Appropriate conversation is a must at the scene of an emergency." Although there are no standards defining what appropriate conversation is, the potential for litigation might exist.

In his book, *Selective Awareness*, Peter Mutke, M.D., describes several cases of iatrogenic communication. (*Iatrogenic* is defined in *Tabor's Cyclopedic Medical Dictionary* as "an abnormal mental or physical condition induced in a patient by effects of treatment by a physician or surgeon. The term implies that such effects could have been avoided by proper and judicious care on the part of the physician.") The cases Dr. Mutke presents involve paramedical personnel and nurses, as well as physicians. In each situation, statements made by rescuers either slowed down or stopped the self-corrective abilities of the patients. The iatrogenic statements were sometimes no more than a careless remark that was overheard or misinterpreted by the patient. In all cases, however, the result was a limited and pessimistic outlook for the recovery of health.

In most instances, the legal principle that all first responders must abide by when performing a rescue is the principle of nonmaleficence. This simply means "to do no further harm." One exception to this principle occurs when a reasonable person could not have foreseen the consequences of a particular action. Similarly, under Good Samaritan laws, rescuers may not be liable "for acts done in good faith." Whether a statement such as "That's the worst hip fracture I've ever seen" or "I don't think this guy is gonna make it" would be construed as reasonable or in good faith would pose an interesting question. Thus the mandate to "avoid inappropriate conversation at the scene of an emergency" may carry with it some legal, if not moral, accountability. But what about legal and moral issues that relate to using positive communication strategies to enhance recovery from medical emergencies? If you are able to direct a patient to stop his or her bleeding with your words and manner, are you stepping outside your boundary?

The "Code of Ethics for Emergency Medical Technicians" adopted by the National Association of Emergency Medical Technicians in 1979 suggests that the answer to this question would be no. It states that the basic responsibility of the EMT is to "conserve life, to alleviate suffering and to promote health." Since there is no injunction against speaking to a patient with confidence, using effective communication skills to offer hope, or suggesting the action of natural healing mechanisms, it would be difficult to imagine a case where you would be liable for directing a patient to stop bleeding, whether or not it worked, *as long as it did not interfere with the standard procedures for treatment.*

Patient
Communication for
First Responders
and EMS Personnel

I Rapport and Expectation

Suggestion does not consist in making an individual
believe what is not true. Suggestion consists in
making something come true by making a person
believe in its possibility.
—J.D. Hadfield

1 | Credibility

The objective of this chapter is to help the student
understand the potential of proper communication with
the person in trauma.

*B*efore words can have a profound effect on someone, they must appear worthy of belief. It is from this sense of credibility that we are motivated to listen and to react. For example, if we were seated at a cafe and a police officer yelled out, "Don't go outside—there's danger!" we would probably respond differently than we would if a young, disruptive child at the next table said the same thing.

Taboo death rituals are an extreme example of the power of words and beliefs. In certain primitive cultures, if a respected shaman puts a death curse on someone, it is likely that the person will actually die. Autopsies of such deaths have revealed an overstimulation of the parasympathetic nervous system. Although it is very unlikely that you or I would be affected by such a directive, people who grow up *believing* in the shaman's power can and do respond accordingly in many instances. The stronger the belief, the more likely the response.

Whenever we are asked or directed to do something, we tend to be more receptive if we perceive the possibility of accomplishing the task. For many years it was believed that no one would ever break the four-minute mile. Though many coaches tried to persuade athletes to run faster and faster, the barrier remained unbroken until one day Jim Ryan managed the "impossible." Within six months, high school and college runners from around the world began running the distance in less than four minutes. Coaches obviously were using the same verbal persuasion as before, but now their words had a sense of credibility.

The placebo effect, taboo death ritual, spontaneous remission of incurable disease, commercial advertising, religious healing, salesmanship, and a host of therapies used in traditional and alternative medicine all give evidence to the power of words when they are presented so as to be worthy of belief.

If a first responder is to be successful when using the directives presented in this text, he must first be perceived by the patient as being credible. The remainder of this chapter provides guidelines and communication strategies for encouraging such credibility. We will begin with a brief historical review describing the power of words as a rapid healing force.

HEALING WITH WORDS: A HISTORICAL PERSPECTIVE

Before the language of words, humans thought only with images. Primitive humans painted the visions of their beliefs on cave walls to share with others in the community and to give them external reality.

Their thoughts and emotions were as images in their minds and could only be expressed through gestures of art, dance, and other ritualistic practices.

The individuals most expressive in these things became the healers of the primitive society. Their ability to get the sick and injured to associate healthful images with ritual worked often enough for others to gain trust for them. Healing shamans were common to preliterate cultures.

As verbal communication developed, words came to function as labels. With labels, objects and experiences could be analyzed and categorized. For example, they were good or bad, safe or dangerous, threatening or nonthreatening, and so on. As the process has evolved, however, there have been errors in judgment, conflicting meanings, and rampant generalizing. New or unlabeled experiences became associated with the categories filed in each person's brain. For example, the experience described by the word *adventure* could be associated with danger, opportunity, challenge, fun, discomfort, and so on. Thus, reaction to the word would depend on the particular association.

In this book you will learn to "unlabel" when communicating directly with an emergency patient. For example, if a patient claims to be an asthmatic or a diabetic, it is helpful to reframe that person's perspective of herself as someone who has a history of suffering from diabetic or asthmatic symptoms. When a paramedic or EMT asks a patient questions, he is not trying to find out what is wrong but is trying to find out what symptoms match a known disease. When an illness is viewed as a process rather than as a part of the person, it is easier to treat or cure it.

As language evolved in this way, medical cures became associated with certain illnesses or injuries. Until relatively recent times, most of the medications that were successful in treating a variety of ills were either pharmacologically inert or based on marginal research. This *placebo effect*, however, has continued to play a significant role in the effect of modern medication. In fact, numerous studies have revealed that the effectiveness of most major medications is due to the placebo effect. In other words, 50 to 60 percent of people given placebos obtain identical results as those given the actual medication.

The placebo effect demonstrates that what we believe and have faith or trust in affects the nervous system more effectively than drugs. In one study, belief even reversed the chemical effect of medication. Patients suffering from chronic nausea were given a "new medicine" to stop their vomiting, and it worked. The medicine, however, was ipecac, a substance that normally induces vomiting.

It may be that the so-called placebo effect is also at work for some surgical procedures. In the 1960s, a physician named Beecher published the results of an experiment relating to the treatment of angina. At that time, an operation referred to as the internal mammary ligation procedure was used to treat angina pain. Internal mammary arteries were tied off to increase blood flow through the coronary artery. The procedure resulted in objectively measured improvements in 98 percent of the cases. Beecher matched patients for age, sex, and duration of illness and performed the operation on half of them. On the other half, he performed a mock operation whereby he prepared them for surgery, anesthetized them, and made an incision in the chest. No further intervention was done with these patients, however. The incision was simply made, then sutured. After recovery, the benefits of the real operation and the mock operation were identical on all objective and subjective measurements, including stress testing.

There have been numerous other studies demonstrating the influence of belief or expectations on surgical procedures. Many have been described in the books listed in the bibliography. Such studies have been reported officially since the advent of modern surgical procedures. For example, in the nineteenth century, several physicians published reports on "painless" surgical operations without the usual high rate of infection and mortality that occurred before the use of chemical anesthesia and sterilization.

The most famous was Dr. James Esdaile, who performed hundreds of such operations while working in India. Most of Dr. Esdaile's patients were natives who believed in the Indian practice of *jar-phoonk*. Jar-phoonk was a ritual that native healers performed on the sick. It consisted of rhythmical stroking and blowing air on a patient until he became relaxed and seemingly distracted from his pain.

James Esdaile's work was neither researched nor welcomed by the medical profession in general. In fact, his practices were treated with much hostility and ridicule by his colleagues. This happened because the orthodox physicians were then trying to free themselves from past connections with magic and religious healing. Struggling to establish an image for themselves as being strictly scientific, the medical profession continued to separate itself from mind-body research.

THE KANSAS EXPERIMENT

This effort to separate traditional physical medicine from psychology has carried over into the field of emergency medicine as well. In 1976,

M. Erik Wright, M.D., Ph.D., an internationally renowned psychologist and psychiatrist, conducted a pioneering research project at an emergency hospital in Kansas. He trained three groups of ambulance attendants to carefully follow several simple communication procedures with emergency patients. First, they were to remove the patient from the crowd as soon as possible to prevent the patient from hearing crowd noise. Second, they were to recite a memorized paragraph designed to calm and reassure the patient and encourage the patient's body systems to work toward survival. (The words and phrasing will be described in later chapters.) The words were to be repeated in a low tone with the paramedic's mouth close to the patient's ear. This was to be done whether or not the patient was unconscious and, of course, like all the procedures in this book, was to be used as an adjunct to standard medical care. Third, no other conversation between the paramedics that could be construed as negative or unrelated to the patient could occur.

The demonstration experiment lasted six months. Treatment outcomes of the patients attended to by the trained paramedics were compared with those of control groups who went about business as usual and who were not so instructed. The results were significant. *The experimental group of patients had more people survive the trip to the hospital and had shorter hospital stays and quicker recovery rates.*

In spite of the remarkable findings of this landmark demonstration, the training program was dropped by the hospital administration when the research funds were exhausted. (The author is currently seeking a grant to replicate this study.) In a presentation before a group of physicians attending an American Society of Clinical Hypnosis Conference, Dr. Wright described the research and his dismay that the training was not continued. Dr. Wright's speech testifies to the importance of proper communication with the emergency patient. His speech is quoted, as follows, in its entirety.

> This study had to do with the training of ambulance attendants who go to a traumatic situation to pick up individuals in various states of tremendous trauma to the body, varying from car accidents, overdoses of drugs, and traumatic events of various kinds, including those not as severely traumatized but nevertheless who cannot bring themselves to the emergency room or hospital situation. These individuals, through the impact of an emergency environment, began to have the terror of survival, the fear of whether or not there is going to be the next moment. And there has been a radical alteration of the life space. The psychological life space has suddenly shrunk so that most of the visually important factors in their life are inconsequential.

Rather, the immediate awareness of their body and the surrounding environment have closed down and the narrowing of
the total psychological functioning has occurred so that there is
an acute responsiveness in some areas and a lack of awareness
in others. This, I think, is important to emphasize besides the
physiological mobilization that has been energized by the trauma. Even shock can be considered a radical mobilization of the
body to preserve essential life functions by placing the body in a
condition of minimum functioning in order to sustain survival
for a given moment. Given these circumstances and some of the
interesting observations of David Cheek and others, we develop
the thesis that in such situations the person's usual critical
responsiveness to the environment has been altered so that
whatever stimuli do reach—whatever language is compre-
hended, whatever communications are received—are often subject to a literal translation and can either aggravate or support
the life systems that are hanging on.

In the experiment, the ambulance attendants were taught a
general statement they were to tell the patient as soon as they
reached the patient:

*The worst is over. We are taking you to the hospital. Everything is
being made ready. Let your body concentrate on repairing itself and
feeling secure. Let your heart, your blood vessels, everything, bring
themselves into a state of preserving your life. Bleed just enough so as to
cleanse the wound, and let the blood vessels close down so that your life
is preserved. Your body weight, your body heat, everything, is being
maintained. Things are being made ready at the hospital for you. We're
getting there as quickly and safely as possible. You are now in a safe
position. The worst is over.*

This kind of rhetoric was repeated in a low-key voice with the
mouth of the attendant close to the patients, whether they were
stuporous, conscious, or unconscious.

The medics were also advised to get quickly away from the
crowd—with all their comments, like "Hey, is that guy gonna
die?" or "Gee, that's a mess," and all of the interventions of
police and others who are so eager to see the "mess" come to a
dramatic end. It's incredible, the language a patient is subject to
at the emergency scene.

Now, this emphasis on the messages being fed in also helped
keep the attendants from talking between themselves, because
they can be the most traumatizing of the patient's exposure to
language as they drive the patient back to the hospital. They

might say, "Man, that's a goner back there," and other things that are said with their focus upon concerns like will they get back in time to catch the last game of the world series and so on. They picked the patient up, put him in a splint, set the IV bottle going with a transfusion, and have called in ahead, and that's it.

The training program taught the attendants to be consciously aware of their responsibility.

It seems absurd to find that such a relatively minor intervention—at least in the demonstration experiences, which lasted six months, comparing the random patients that were picked up by the experimental crews (there were three crews) with the patients that were picked up by the nontrained control crews—could make such a difference in, first, the number who were not dead on arrival but who survived the trip, those who were sustained and able to be treated, and those who had a quicker recovery rate. Now the fact that this demonstration was statistically valid doesn't mean that the process of training was adopted, because once the demonstration funds ran out, nothing else was done about it. That's quite independent. But from the point of view of a demonstration of a radical shift, which took into account that in a state of severe traumatization there is still (as long as life persists) a communication system. There is still a focus of attention where the critical state of the patient has caused an uncritical acceptance of options. The support framework of language becomes a significant contributor to the health care management of the individual. It is so absurdly simple that you become, at least I become, terribly distressed, because you can't budge administrative organizations to initiate this kind of processing. During the training the [paramedics] themselves become the proselytizers and we had difficulty in keeping them from spoiling the experiment and teaching the others. So, the environment of treatment begins with the first initial contact between any of the medical viable personnel to the very last terminal relationship when the patient leaves the hospital. We need to understand the need for a structure of language which is supportive and recognizes the translation of comments.

Since Dr. Wright's death in 1981 and prior to the publication of this book, relatively little has been done to teach these principles of patient communication to first responders. One exception is a video, "Effective Communication with the Sick and Injured," available through Hope Counseling, 205 San Marin Drive, Suite 2, Novato,

CA, 94945. For general medical self-help, however, the similar concepts of imagery and belief are a part of most books now published on the subject.

HOW WORDS INFLUENCE HEALING

When we see with our eyes, what we ultimately perceive relates to a photochemical reaction that triggers nerve impulses conducted to the brain's cerebral cortex. This area of the brain decodes the impulses via image responsive chemicals that create our perception. Whether or not the images are meaningful is determined by learned experience.

All we need in order to experience an image and an associated perception is for the appropriate neuronal pathways to fire. It does not matter whether they fire because of stimulation to the retina or other sense organs, or because of an internal image, such as dream, imagination, or memory image.

Medical science has been aware of this fact since the 1920s, when American physician and physiologist Edmund Jacobson did experiments proving that, when people imagined themselves involved in an action like running or swimming, the muscles in their body associated with that action contracted in amounts that could be measured with special equipment. Further research has shown that virtually every cell in the body can be influenced by images held in the mind's eye. Through the pathways between the cerebral cortex, where images are stored, and the automatic nervous system, such images can control

sweating

blood pressure

blood vessel expansion and contraction

flushing

goose pimpling

pain response

heart rate and force of contraction

respiratory rate

dryness of mouth

immune response

bowel motility

smooth muscle tension

glandular secretions

inflammatory response

blood coagulation

allergic response

rate of healing

dermatitis

emotional reactions

and so on.

During times of fear, emotional factors combine with old belief systems to create images that may influence one or more of the above functions negatively. The same factors, however, can make an individual highly receptive toward new directions from someone who is perceived as a trusted leader or authority figure.

This process seems to occur in animals as well. On one hand, frightened animals do not do well in captivity and often die. On the other hand, even frightened wild animals can be extremely trusting of very confident and caring humans, allowing themselves to be handled or cared for.

Perhaps this increased receptivity is a natural protective mechanism common to all species. In times of confusion it allows for quick responses to the directions of herd or tribal leaders. If this is a primitive survival function, it makes sense that it is initiated in the limbic system, the oldest part of the brain. The major function of the limbic system is to compare incoming stimuli from the body with instructions programmed by previous experiences. It interacts with the cerebral cortex in analyzing data.

A component of the limbic system is the *amygdala*. Here emotional responses are triggered when incoming stimuli do not fit expected patterns. If something new and unexpected happens, like a medical emergency, it will send out impulses that trigger the release of hormones in an effort to prepare the body for fight or flight.

Unfortunately, most of the programming of past experiences that directs the activity of the amygdala consists of old patterns that were programmed during infancy and early childhood when we were not sufficiently conscious to clearly evaluate the addictions of our parents, teachers, and others. Because these instructions still reside in our biocomputers, in most emergency situations (in our culture) we end up doing that which violates our first survival interests. In most cases, neither fight nor flight is an appropriate reaction.

Fortunately, fear, stress, and confusion also increase the potential for adaptation by increasing activity in the brain's image center. Many researchers believe that such image-making activity occurs in the right hemisphere of the brain. In his book, *The Healing Mind*, Dr. Irving Oyle refers to studies conducted by Dr. Julian Jaynes, author of *The Origin of Consciousness in the Breakdown of the Bicameral Mind*. He states, "Dr. Jaynes suggested that right-brained, holographic activity is precipitated by stress. My own clinical observations seem to confirm his hypothesis. The more acute the suffering, the stronger the stimulus for salvation or compensating image production by the right hemisphere."

It is known that the image-responsive chemicals in the right brain somehow trigger the secretion of hormones, including neuro-hormones, that control the pituitary and endocrine systems, adrenalin, noradrenalin, and endorphins. Ultimately, these hormones and others are involved in the regulation of the sympathetic and parasympathetic nervous system. Language centers in the left brain provide a mode of access for the description and interpretation of images. However, the specific relationship between words and images is not understood. Words not only describe images, they also create them.

We do know, however, that there are at least three times when image-responsive centers in the brain become active enough to affect physiological processes that can enhance recovery from medical emergencies. These three times are as follows:

1. Following the acceptance of a belief. Images follow beliefs. When belief is formed, the mind begins to accept images that relate to it. Placebos are an example of this. The more a patient believes in the rescuer, the more likely the rescuer's words will cause the creation of effective healing images.

2. While involved in passive concentration. Image activity also increases when active, analytical thinking slows down and is replaced with focused attention. This focus is fundamental to such things as hypnosis, self-hypnosis, biofeedback, meditation, yoga, autogenics, visualization, Zen, and so on. This kind of concentration requires training and practice.

3. During periods of emotional excitement, emotions prepare the body to defend itself against harm. Fear increases the ability to run away, while anger increases aggressive capabilities. As we have mentioned, however, when neither fight nor flight are appropriate,

the emotional state opens up receptivity to the suggestions of a trusted authority figure. This partially explains the power a charismatic, trusted individual can have over people during times of stress. History is full of illustrations where such leaders have persuaded people to do remarkable things, good or bad.

BODY LANGUAGE

It is important to remember, as you study the communication strategies in the following chapter, that the delivery of words is as important as the words alone while attempting to influence the patient's images. Dr. Noel Burch is coauthor (with Dr. Thomas Gordon) of *Teacher Effectiveness Training*. Using Dr. Ray L. Birdwhistell's research from the University of Pennsylvania, Dr. Burch says that, when a person is communicating, 70 percent of his message is sent by his body language, 23 percent by the tone or inflection of his voice, and only 7 percent by the words that are used. Of course, this research was not done with frightened emergency patients, who often cannot see their rescuers clearly during rescue operations. If it had been, it is likely that tone or inflection would have been the most significant. In any case, the importance of nonverbal communication cannot be overstated.

Many books have been written on the subject of body language, but all you need to know as a first responder is to be confident, sincere, and caring. If you concentrate on being nonjudgmental, if you remain relaxed, and if you make eye contact with your patient when you speak, your body language will join the force of your words and techniques to send the appropriate messages.

TRUE OR FALSE?

1. Protective mechanisms in the body can overreact to injury and illness.

2. Words and images can influence autonomic nervous system functions.

3. Dr. Wright's Kansas experiment showed that the words spoken by paramedics had no significant effect on treatment outcome.

4. Fear increases receptivity to the directions of a trusted authority figure.

5. Body language is not as important as words.

The greatest thing in all education is to make the nervous system our ally instead of our enemy.
—William James

2 | Confidence

The objective of this chapter is to teach the student how to project confidence at the emergency scene.

THE FIRST STEP

If a rescuer's words are to be perceived with a sufficient degree of credibility, then they must be spoken with confidence. This is the first step toward preparing the patient to accept directives that can mobilize health-stabilizing responses.

In many cases, emergency patients will believe a professional rescuer simply because of the official uniform. However, first responders may not always be in uniform; some injuries prevent a patient from seeing her rescuers; and occasionally a uniform triggers distrust and resentment in a patient. Furthermore, a patient may quickly lose confidence in even a uniformed medic if the latter's words and manner are inappropriate or are lacking in confidence. Emergency patients are also very sensitive to touch. If you are worried or pessimistic, do not touch the patient until you feel sure of yourself and what you can do. It is therefore necessary to learn how to project confidence at the emergency scene.

DEVELOPING CONFIDENCE

The following sections will help you to develop and project the confidence you need at the site of an emergency. Use these sections as guidelines.

Know Yourself and Have Faith in Your Abilities

To maintain confidence amidst crisis, you must have faith in yourself. This means believing in your ability to effectively communicate with the patient and to use your first aid skills and knowledge *as best you can*. Such a belief comes from knowing your strengths, acknowledging your weaknesses (while working to improve them), and going all out to achieve what you can for the patient. This willingness to face any problem within the range of your capabilities provides for the experiences necessary to develop a confident attitude at the emergency scene.

It is important to be realistic about your strengths and weaknesses while developing such a confident belief in your abilities. If you hold back at the emergency scene, letting others do work you yourself could do, you miss opportunities to succeed and build confidence. If you try to do more than your abilities allow, attempting to overcompensate for a lack of confidence, you will make too many mistakes and this will decrease your confidence further.

Also, do not emphasize confidence in a particular skill or ability or you will tend to show it off at the expense of a true total confidence, and the patient will *not* respond to your suggestions (though they may be impressed with your particular skills). Do not advertise.

Analyze—do not criticize. To learn your strengths and weaknesses and develop confidence, make a list of them and determine which ones you can improve. Run reviews are a good way to help with this list. Then focus on the strengths and go over them in your mind on your way to the call.

Improve Fitness, Training, and Equipment

Physical fitness breeds confidence. A fit rescuer has the strength and stamina to handle difficult and strenuous calls. He has reserves of energy that can help with clear thinking and calm communication with the victim. Continual training in medical and rescue procedures is also important, as is having faith in one's equipment.

Conquer Fear

Certainly, fear is a reasonable emotion to expect a first responder to have when initially confronting a potentially hazardous emergency scene. It should serve as a warning to carefully assess the situation—act appropriately to avoid danger if possible. Once fear has served this function, however, there is no longer any need to hold on to it. Doing so will cause unnecessary stress and will detract from your ability to project confidence to the frightened patient.

Besides fear of physical harm, first responders are often fearful of psychological or "ego" harm. They are afraid to say the wrong thing, to use the incorrect first aid procedure, or to appear foolish while using the special communication strategies described in this text. They may also be afraid of legal consequences relative to helping a medical emergency patient.

Whatever the particular stimulus for fear, the first step in keeping this emotion in *motion*, thereby moving beyond it, is to consciously reason with yourself about the actual risk and benefit involved. Perhaps as much as 98 percent of what we fear will happen, will not. It is reasonable to risk 2 percent for the sake of helping another human being or even for the sake of personal growth. When we stop wrestling with fear and use reason to determine a basis for action in the face of it, the fear will disappear. If you wrestle with it, you will pin it to you, and your patients will know it. But when you instead concentrate on the skills, the work, the action, the task, and the needs of the patient, new positive emotions will follow the nature of your concentration. Then the patient will believe in you. (Note: It is important to be aware of the difference between fear and arousal, though the physiological responses are similar. It is natural to have an increase in adrenalin when involved in emergency rescue and care. An increased arousal level will not be conveyed as fear to the patient.)

Many first responders utilize humor to overcome fear. This is an excellent approach, but care must be taken not to appear insensitive to the patient. Later we will discuss techniques for the use of humor with patients to reduce stress and fear.

Monitor Emotional Reactions

To maintain the positive transference of confidence that is fundamental to the optimal effect of words or treatment outcome, the first-aider must constantly be aware of her own emotional reactions. Many emergency scenes will present numerous factors that could easily trigger such emotions as anger, disgust, hate, horror, or sadness. The EMT, or first responder, must learn to quickly move beyond such emotions when they arise so they do not disrupt the flow of confident communication.

Although such composure can be achieved with the guidelines described in "Conquer Fear" above, do not expect to be able to completely transcend these human feelings. Unlike fear, which is an emotion to prompt appropriate action and which can be overcome when such action is taken, other emotions will ultimately require release as well. The time for this is after the call, when all the emotions should be ventilated and discussed with other understanding individuals. In extreme cases, a professional counselor should be consulted.

Focus on the Patient—Not Yourself

In all forms of effective communication, from writing to public speaking, a basic rule is that the speaker thinks of the audience's needs, not his own. When using the techniques and strategies presented in this book to develop rapport, build expectations, and give powerful healing directives, sincere concern for the patient must far outweigh ego considerations. If you worry about how you are going to sound, how you will appear in the eyes of others, or whether or not you will be successful, the chances are that you will not convey sufficient confidence to the patient. Remember that emergency patients become highly aware of their surroundings and will be able to tune in to the degree of sincerity being expressed by those around them.

Control Extraverbal Signals

In addition to the semantics of language, a patient perceives messages from nonverbal, intraverbal and extraverbal signals. Although this occurs during normal communication, the alternative state of consciousness of a frightened emergency patient creates an intensified focus of attention. As a result, such an individual is quick to perceive subtleties of communication that may not be obvious to you. Thus, take care to control the following:

- Nonverbal gestures such as facial expressions, shoulder shrugs, clenched fists, and so on.

- Intraverbal intonations of words. This relates to emphasis placed on certain words. For example, there is a difference between saying, "We're going to get you *out* of there," and "We're *going* to get you out of there." The former infers a sense of urgency about getting the patient out, which could be a frightening perception to her. The second emphasizes a sense of confidence that there is no doubt the patient is *going* to be extricated.

- Extraverbal implications of words and gestures. Certain dialogue can have tacit meanings that could cause resistance. For example, "Why don't you lie down?" tacitly implies a criticism that might be interpreted, "You fool—why are you standing up?" A better phrase would be, "Would you be more comfortable lying down?"

Frequently a first responder manages to speak with confidence but inadvertently reveals concern, worry, or fear to the patient with his body language. Since most first responders are going to have such thoughts in many instances, it is important to learn how to prevent this unintentional communication.

Actors, courtroom lawyers, diplomats, negotiators, and salespeople have all learned both to control their own nonverbal cues and to read them in others. They have learned this with training and practice in voice tone and inflection as well as in control of facial expression, use of hands, posture, and so on.

The best way to develop this control is with simulation and feedback sessions. Simulate an emergency situation with a pretend patient and an observer. Administer first aid and communicate using the guidelines and scripts contained in this text. Although it will be difficult to reproduce the anxieties and concerns of an actual emergency, try your best to get into the role. A degree of performance anxiety will also help challenge your confidence.

The job of the observer is to note the ways in which you convey a lack of confidence. Note the appropriate criticisms, and practice again with different movements, postures, and voice tones until you are able to hide any cues that might convey anxiety or lack of confidence. (You might begin with a confident, assuring smile.)

Develop a Good Relaxation Response

The ability to project confidence is related to the ability to relax. The latter requires practice. On a daily basis you should spend fifteen to thirty minutes or more using some form of relaxation or meditation. A variety of alternatives exist, such as autogenic training, Transcendental Meditation, Tai Chi, and yoga. The technique developed by Dr. Edmund Jacobson in the 1920s is also an excellent method.

This simply involves making yourself comfortable in an area where you are not likely to be disturbed. Then, beginning with the feet and working up the body to the face and scalp, tighten the muscles, then relax them until the entire body is in a state of relaxation.

As you become accustomed to the type of relaxation response you choose, the state of relaxation will occur more and more rapidly until you can enter it spontaneously, even at an emergency scene. Although your arousal level will maintain sufficient adrenalin to help you perform, the ability to relax will help you calm and reassure the patient.

Rehearse Your Techniques

Once you have developed your own style of communication utilizing the scripts and guidelines presented later, you should practice them like an actor memorizing lines.

This includes both active practice, as in a simulation, and mental rehearsal. The best time for mental rehearsal (visualization of yourself communicating at an emergency) is during a relaxation session. Although each actual emergency situation will be unique, you will easily be able to modify the learned scripts to fit the emergency event.

Be in the Now

Many philosophers refer to the point of power being in the present. We can focus on the present moment, without thoughts of past or future; we can concentrate exclusively on what is happening around us. Although preplanning and practice contribute to our effectiveness at the emergency scene, do not dwell on potential calls in between practice sessions. Remain in "the now" and you will have all the confidence you ever need.

EXERCISES

1. Make a list of your strengths and weaknesses when confronting an emergency crisis.

2. Describe a situation where a physically fit rescuer would be better prepared to handle an emergency than would be a physically unfit one.

3. Explain the difference between extraverbal, intraverbal and non-verbal signals.

4. Describe the Jacobsonian relaxation response.

5. Tell how a paramedic could be mentally in the future or past during a rescue, rather than in the present.

I must take leave to tell you that the medical man who has not studied the laws of mind as well as matter, and how they act and react to each other, is very unfit for practicing his profession, either with credit to himself or advantage to his patient.
—James Braid

3 | Rapport

This chapter's primary goal is to teach strategies that will develop trust between the patient and the first responder.

THE BRIDGE OF COMMUNICATION

Patients best respond to words when they have trust in or rapport with the speaker. This rapport supports hope for the future and thus a willingness to consider alternatives to reinterpretations of the situation. It decreases physical tension and the defensive posture that increases debilitating stress. It opens pathways that can mobilize natural healing capabilities.

Certainly the projection of confidence is a prerequisite to positive rapport. Also, the wearing of an official uniform can contribute. However, in many cases, skillful communication is required to gain and maintain rapport. This chapter will present a variety of such communication strategies and techniques.

Before reviewing such approaches, it should be noted that one aspect of rapport cannot be taught. This relates to that instant rapport that can exist between individuals. Sometimes it can be negative and sometimes, positive. When it is positive, rapport and trust are automatic, as though the result of a long and sacred friendship.

It should also be noted that it may be impossible to gain positive rapport when the patient is intoxicated or has taken drugs. Although such people *may* respond extremely well to your words, it is also possible that you will not be able to get their attention. In any case, when helping someone so affected, it is important to continue trying to establish rapport.

ACHIEVING RAPPORT

As with the strategies presented in Chapter 2 for gaining confidence, the following sections offer guidelines for achieving rapport with the emergency patient. Use one or more of these strategies when attempting to establish this necessary positive rapport.

Give Yourself a Proper Introduction

Your first opportunity to establish a positive rapport with a patient is when you arrive at the scene and make initial contact. Rather than starting medical treatment without saying anything (as is often done), take a moment to introduce yourself.

Since the initial contact is at the peak of a first responder's anxiety level, it is important to take a moment to gather confidence and decide a plan of action before speaking to or touching the patient. Then, while beginning extrication or medical treatment, or just before so doing, explain who you are and what you aim to do. Remember to speak slowly and clearly to the patient.

When possible, it is helpful to find out the name of the patient before you are in her presence. Knowing her name ahead of time allows you to address the patient more intimately at the outset. Asking someone else the patient's name in the presence of a conscious patient is not a good way to start. Doing so tends to be a little demeaning and confirms the sense of helplessness the person is already feeling. If you cannot get the name from someone else, without the patient overhearing, then it is best to ask her name directly. (If the patient is about your age or younger, use the first name. If the patient is a senior, it may be more respectful to refer to them as Mr. or Mrs.)

Generally, most introductions will be similar for you from one time to another. It may therefore be helpful if you memorize one that feels comfortable. You can then adapt it according to each different situation. The following examples will give you an idea of how to construct an effective introduction. Modify one of these to suit your own style of communication.

Introduction to a Conscious Patient Whose Name Is Known

> Hello, John. I'm Don. I'm an EMT with the County fire department, and I'm here to help you. OK? Good. We'll have you out of here soon.

> Mary, can you hear me? Good. I know you're uncomfortable, but the worst is over now. I'm an EMT, and we're here to help you.

> Bill, my name is Don, and I can help you. The worst is over, but I need you to help me as best you can. Will you do that? Good.

Notice that, in all three examples, several objectives were met.

First, each patient was addressed with his or her own name. This provides recognition and familiarity. Second, each patient was asked a question. This gives a sense of control to the patient at the outset. Third, you have introduced yourself as someone who can help; and fourth, a sense that the future is hopeful is suggested.

After introducing yourself in such a way as to meet these four objectives, it is usually helpful to inject some degree of humor into the situation. This can be done best by identifying a problem obvious to the patient so as to get him or her to acknowledge the ridiculous aspect of it. For example, "Gee, Bill, I don't think your car will sell for blue book now," or "Well, Mary, I hope you weren't planning on wearing this dress out to dinner tomorrow night," or "I'll bet you can think of something you'd rather be doing than this."

Of course, a great deal of tact and sensitivity must be used when being humorous at the emergency scene. If you are sincere and caring, however, any effort at humor will usually be helpful. If there is no positive response to your humor, ask the patient "Have you been under any emotional stress prior to the accident?" In many instances, an injury or an accident causes a person to focus on other negative stresses in their life until these cannot be separated from the accident. When you ask this question, the patient has the opportunity to make the separation and thus get on with the process of survival.

David Cheek asked this question to a patient brought into the emergency room when he was on duty. The patient was a forty-two-year-old unmarried woman who had been found unconscious on her living room floor in a pool of blood. When she arrived at the hospital, she appeared to be unconscious, and her skin was cold and mottled on appearance. Her respiration was shallow and rapid; her pulse rate was 140.

Dr. Cheek leaned over to her and asked, "Have you been under any emotional stress lately?" This was the first remark anyone had said to her. She opened her eyes and answered, "Oh, I'm so ashamed. I've been going with my friend now for two years, and I had intercourse with him last night." Dr. Cheek laughed and said, "For goodness sake, why did you wait so long?" At this point, color returned to the woman's cheeks, she smiled and asked Dr. Cheek not to tell her roommate, and her pulse dropped to 100.

If there is no one to tell you the patient's name, then ask it directly, regardless of how severe the injury or illness. If the patient cannot or will not answer you, tell her that that's quite all right, then continue treating the patient and talking to her. Remember that, *even if the patient is unconscious, it is very important to tell her what you are going to do before you do it.* Unconscious patients can, at some level, hear all the words that are spoken in their presence. (More will be discussed about this in Chapter 12, "Cardiovascular Emergencies.")

Introduction to a Conscious Patient Whose Name Is Unknown

Hello, I'm Jim Brown. I'm a paramedic. Can you tell me your first name? [Patient answers with name.] Good, Bill, we're going to check you over now and help make you better.

In giving you his or her name, the patient begins to regain a little sense of control. In hearing the name called back, a sense of familiarity and comfort is had.

Introduction to an Unconscious Patient Who Is Breathing

> Hello, Richard. I'm Don and there is someone else here named Frank. We're both paramedics, and we're here to help you. Go ahead and leave your eyes closed for a while longer while we take your blood pressure.

Introduction to an Unconscious Patient Who Is Not Breathing

> Hello, Jean. My name is Don and I'm a paramedic. I'm here to help you. I'm going to lift your jaw and tilt your head back to make it easier for you to breathe. You're going to be all right.

Show Respect for the Patient

Respect is a two-way street. If you show respect for patients, they will return the feeling twofold and are likely to do what you say.

Unfortunately, professional prehospital care personnel often present a superior attitude that tends to demean the patient. Although an authoritarian approach is sometimes called for and will be discussed later, it is usually preferable to treat patients with utmost consideration. This includes a respect for their modesty, their intelligence, their concerns, and their potential ability to cope.

This also means respect for the patient's ability to communicate. The patient should not be the last one to have input about his medical problem. When possible, simply asking the patient to describe the problem will build rapport. Similarly, letting the patient tell you in what position he is most comfortable or what need he can identify will help develop a sense of mutual respect.

Using the same language as the patient also tends to promote trust, if it is done without mockery. If you talk to a construction worker the same way you talk to a college professor, or vice versa, you will not achieve optimal rapport. Trust is also threatened if you use baby talk with the elderly or if you are less than truthful.

One good way to gain trust quickly is to use the patient's proper name. Use your judgment.

Show a Sincere Concern for the Patient

A respect for someone's rights, privileges, and abilities is slightly separate from a sincere concern for her welfare. The latter, however, will also do much to gain rapport. If an emergency patient is convinced that your intentions are totally aimed at her well-being, the trust required for effective communication becomes more likely.

Having such concern for a patient who is a stranger may not be automatic for a first responder, professional or otherwise. In some situations, the emergency patient may even appear disgusting or unworthy. Rescuers often go through the motions of emergency care without really caring. Such treatment diminishes rapport and the potential for effective communication.

Cultivating sincerity for the well-being of medical emergency patients requires a personal commitment to basic humanitarian objectives. For the professional, this commitment should be reviewed regularly. The original desire to help others that brings people into emergency medical service (EMS) can become calloused after many calls. Duty is not the same as sincerity. The most proficient medical treatment without the additional power of effective communication falls short of what should be accomplished for the patient.

If the patient is a loved one or a personal friend, it is important for the rescuer not to show overconcern for his welfare. This could be misinterpreted as worry and could diminish positive rapport to a point where directives are disregarded.

Talk in the Patient's Language

If it can be done naturally, without obvious effort or mockery, talking to a person in his own language facilitates trust. This, of course, includes speaking a foreign language when necessary, but refers primarily to the style of conversation. Learning the lingo and slang of different population groups can also be an asset.

Another aspect of a personal language relates to a person's personality. If you listen carefully to what a patient is saying and how she is saying it, you can more easily relate to her and thus, she to you. If the person conveys a sense of courage, talk to her frankly and indirectly acknowledge her strength. If someone conveys a sense of humor, do not be humorless in your approach.

Often a style of communication can be determined by observing the clothing of a patient. For example, if a woman is wearing unique, handmade jewelry, she has told you that she is unique and creative. In this case it would be easier for you to gain rapport by acknowledging this in your communication. For example, you might say to such a person, "What I'm going to ask you may seem a little unusual, but I want you to hold the IV while I check out your leg." Asking them to do anything offbeat that would not be harmful will help you speak their language.

Very simple phrases are often sufficient to put you on a patient's language level. For example, to an army general you might say, "This is the routine thing to do"; to a high school freshman, "Hang loose while I do this"; to a well-groomed man in a business suit, "The most efficient thing we can do now is this."

Talking in the patient's language might also mean being in agreement with them. For example, if a patient tells you that he does not trust people in uniform, you might reply, "Sometimes people in uniform can be difficult to get along with, but of course that isn't always true. In spite of my uniform, I want you to know that I am here to help you." By initially tending to agree with the patient, and then gradually modifying his defenses, you can begin to build on the rapport you gained with the agreement.

Maintain a Proper Balance of Power

Rapport is a delicate matter at the emergency scene. A patient monitors her trust carefully. If the "hidden observer" in the patient's mind perceives a threat, rapport is quickly lost. Maintaining a proper balance of power is one way to keep this hidden observer content.

Balance of power relates to the degree of control that is shared between the patient and the rescuer. This is different in every case. Some patients will need more control, some will need less. Furthermore, the degree of power may fluctuate back and forth during a single case.

Determining the balance of power is an experimental process. It is usually best to begin by offering the patient the majority of control and then gradually usurping it as necessary. For example, you might ask the patient to hold an ice pack on an injury, hence acknowledging his power. If, however, the patient does not respond positively to this, the balance of power should shift more to you. If you feel the patient has a high degree of control in a situation, you might ask him to handle pain by saying, "You seem to be handling yourself well; can you stay just as relaxed as you are right now while I take your blood pressure?"

If, on the other hand, the patient does not seem to be in much control, it would be preferable to say, "I know you are uncomfortable, but I want you to listen to me carefully. We are going to do everything we can to help make you more comfortable." In this latter situation, the power shift to the rescuer would be a more effective way to help with the patient's pain.

Some degree of power should always be given to the patient, regardless of how much he is willing to take. An easy way to ensure that this is being done is to *always tell the patient what you are going to do before you do it.* For example, if you are about to put on a blood pressure cuff, you must first say, "I'm going to go ahead and put the blood pressure cuff on your arm so we can get a reading. There you go, now I'm going to put some air in it, and you'll notice it becoming more snug."

Occasionally, you will find that a "one-down" position of power will build more rapport than a "one-up" position. An emergency patient is already feeling out of control of her environment and may not need further insult as a result of being treated as an inferior being. If you reveal your own weakness, she may feel less threatened. For example, "Bear with me, if you would. I'm a little slow when it comes to getting a good medical history. I want to make sure to ask all the right questions." This kind of exchange can help not only to iron out any potential power struggle but also to establish a first-name basis between you.

Make Realistic Statements

When you lose credibility in the eyes of the patient, you lose rapport. It is therefore important to make statements that are realistic. An example of an unrealistic sentence might be, "There's nothing to worry about," when told to a patient who is uninsured and who just crashed an expensive car into a parked school bus. Although seemingly improbable directives will ultimately be effective at this stage of communication, care must be taken to keep sentences realistic.

This rule is especially critical when dealing with children. For instance, if you were to tell a child that his cut didn't look too bad and that it couldn't hurt too much, you might instantly lose rapport and have difficulty both in patient management and treatment outcome. A more appropriate sentence would be, "Wow, look at that cut—I'll bet that hurts." With this approach, the child would acknowledge that you know what you are doing because you indeed understand how he or she feels. Then you can begin to change the child's feelings.

Use Feedback Strategy to Gain Rapport

A good communication tool is to be a keen observer. A successful trial lawyer or salesperson, for example, is able to note the needs and concerns of her audience. By addressing such concerns before the listener consciously conveys the information, the speaker presents herself as someone with special insight—someone who should be trusted. Professional con men have mastered the feedback strategy to such a degree that, within a very short time, they can cause their targets to entrust them with their life savings.

By being observant of your patient, you can also demonstrate this rapport-building "special insight." Here are just a few examples of feedback strategies.

Situation:

The rescuer arrives at a traffic accident, to find a seriously injured twenty-four-year-old female lying in the street. She is conscious and extremely frightened. Within five minutes he has completed primary and secondary surveys and all possible field treatment. The patient appears less frightened, and her pulse has lowered. Then the sounds of ambulance and police sirens appear as they approach the scene from about a half mile out. The rescuer's observations of the patient signal that the sirens will trigger increased anxiety, so he says, "Well, here comes some more help. I know the sirens sound frightening, but they do keep us from getting stuck in traffic."

Having addressed her concern, seemingly before she herself consciously displayed it, the rescuer will have increased rapport while at the same time reducing her anxiety.

Situation:

A forty-two-year-old male has suffered burns from an oil tank explosion, and the rescuer has placed an oxygen mask on his face and is administering oxygen. While the rescuer is adjusting the liter flow, he notices the patient start to bring his hand up to the mask and slightly turn his head. The rescuer realizes that the man is about to be bothered by the confining structure on his face. Before the patient's anxiety builds and he tries to remove the mask, the rescuer says, "You might be a little bothered by the mask. Most people are at first. But if you just concentrate on that nice, fresh, relaxing flow of oxygen, you will notice how much more comfortable it can become."

With this sentence the rescuer will have gained sufficient rapport with the patient to immediately follow with a directive such as, "But, if you just concentrate on . . . ." As the patient actually becomes comfortable with the mask, he further acknowledges the rescuer's "special insight."

Another way to successfully use the feedback strategy is to simply repeat what the patient has told you afterwards. The patient may or may not remember that he gave you the information. In either case, trust in you will be increased when the patient hears you state what he believes to be true. Your statement can be made to another paramedic or can be fed back to the patient. The statements can include the patient's stated symptoms, complaints, concerns, desires, and so on. They can also relate to observation of the patient. For example, if the patient swallows, you might say, "You might notice how soothing it feels to swallow."

Congratulate Patient on Positive Responses

When you commend a patient for following your directions, you enhance rapport with that person. We are accustomed to bonding with people who congratulate us, whether they have been teachers, parents, coaches, or friends. Do not be overly patronizing with your praise, unless talking to a small child. Simply saying, "That's good," will usually be sufficient. For example, if you ask the patient to take a deep breath and she does, simply say, "Good." When using this approach to specifically develop rapport, be sure to give some directives that you know the patient can and will follow.

Join In with Patient, then Reframe

Another strategy for assuring positive rapport with a patient is to initially "join in" with that person in his complaint. This could mean an agreement or even a mimicking or sharing of the presenting signs or symptoms. Joining in works especially well with a patient who would be likely to turn off to a rescuer who attempted to directly stop or change his destructive behavior. In most cases such patients will be highly emotional. This strategy is also very effective with asthma attacks and hyperventilation, or panic attacks.

To join in with a patient in respiratory distress, begin mimicking his breathing rate and rhythm while saying, "I know . . . how difficult . . . it is . . . for you to get an easy . . . full breath . . . ." (For an asthma patient this can be done while preparing to administer oxygen.)

At this point, while your breathing rate is in rhythm with the patient's, gradually begin to slow down the rate and watch how the patient will now start to follow *your* lead. As you do so, say, "But notice how much . . . easier . . . it is becoming to take a nice, easy, full, relaxing breath." When the patient begins to breathe normally, congratulate him by saying, "That's good."

First responders often need to calm a hysterical patient or an emotionally out-of-control relative. Joining-in strategies can be very helpful in such situations. Simply acknowledging the distraught person's feelings can have a noticeable calming effect. Thus, instead of saying, "It's okay. He's going to be fine. Just calm down," say "You're real scared, but we're going to take good care of him." This approach tends to build instant rapport and makes the person more compliant to subsequent instruction.

Divert Attention from Injuries

Whenever an action or statement of the rescuer actually increases the comfort of the patient, rapport is enhanced. Diversion is a relatively easy way to accomplish this. When the patient's attention can be distracted from her problem or pain, there is an actual decrease in the discomfort until her attention again focuses on the problem. When the diversion is a direct result of listening to the rescuer, the patient will associate the temporary relief with the rescuer's words and rapport is developed.

A variety of questions and directions can be used to get the patient to direct attention to something apart from her chief complaint. Asking the person's age, having her pay attention to the blood pressure cuff, or involving her in the treatment of a minor complaint—all can serve the purpose.

An excellent way to achieve diversion is with the secondary survey. Ask the patient to tell you the degree of discomfort felt when you press on a part of her body. Then, intentionally begin to press on areas you know are not involved with pain or injury. As the patient's attention focuses on these places and the pressure of your hand, she will momentarily forget the main injury. Subconsciously, this relief will be associated with your words, and this will create a positive rapport, or *transference*.

The statement, I'll bet you can imagine someplace else you'd rather be right now, followed by the question, asked matter-of-factly, What would you be doing if you could be doing your favorite thing? can be very effective in diverting the patient's attention away from pain and discomfort. Very often, the patient will allow her imagination to take her to a warm beach in Mexico or to a hammock under the trees. More will be discussed about such imagery when we discuss expectations and directives.

Obtain a Direct Contract with the Patient

Hello. My name is John. I'm a paramedic, and I'm here to help you. *Will* you do what I say?

This is an example of a direct contract for rapport. If the patient agrees, this may be all that is needed for him to follow subsequent directives designed to influence critical autonomic functions.

Most of the above communication approaches for achieving rapport have been indirect strategies. In some cases, rapport can be obtained with a direct contract at the outset of care. A direct contract is best attempted when the first responder feels very confident and the patient appears to be very receptive. Otherwise, a rejection of the contract may temporarily block rapport. It should be noted, however, that failure to achieve the direct contract initially is not at all a serious setback. The use of the indirect strategies will soon put you back on track.

It is recommended that you study the preceding rapport strategies so that they can be used spontaneously throughout any emergency rescue or patient treatment. When positive rapport is easily achieved with one technique, use of the others will help maintain it. When a particular technique does not work for you, continue trying with it and others until rapport is gained or until the patient is no longer in your care. Even if rapport is not gained until after field treatment has been given and the patient is about to be put in an ambulance, its eventual achievement will allow you to offer a departing directive that could significantly affect future treatment outcome.

It should also be noted that rapport with a patient might first be gained by a bystander before you arrive. Someone in the crowd surrounding the emergency scene might yell, "Oh my God, that person is going to die if he isn't moved away from the car!" This may have been said with such conviction, sincerity, and authority as to create rapport sufficient for the patient to believe in the statement. Thus, until you are able to establish rapport, it is helpful to keep people in the crowd from interfering when possible.

TRANSFERRING RAPPORT

If you are a first responder and have gained a positive rapport with the emergency patient, it can be troubling to watch your patient being transferred to the care of others who do not have good rapport and who make no effort to acquire it. To help prevent this from happening, you can transfer your rapport to the next tier of support.

The EMS tier of support is as follows:

First responder (citizen, fire department, etc.)

Paramedic

Emergency room physician

There are two parts to the transfer. The first is a statement to the patient that gives your personal endorsement to the next EMS provider.

Tom, this is Bill. He's a paramedic. He will build on the care I have begun. He's going to check you over and might even ask some of the same questions I did. You're in good hands with him.

The second part in the transfer requires that you inform the next provider that you have gained a positive rapport with the patient and that the patient has been responding positively to your directives. (See Chapter 5 "General Directives.") You can make this statement in the presence of the patient if you choose or if it is necessary to do so anyway. If the patient hears what you are saying, it will only serve to reinforce the statement.

Bill, this is Tom. Tom's complaining of discomfort in his lower right abdomen. I've written down his vitals and response levels for you. Tom is doing very well. I'm sure he'll do as well for you as he's done for me.

In many instances, especially if you have been with the patient for a long time before assistance arrives, you may have given the patient a particular directive that is working very effectively. For example, "Whenever you take a deep breath, your discomfort will lessen." Be sure to share this directive with the next medical provider so she can repeat or reinforce the directive when needed.

TRUE OR FALSE?

1. To maintain rapport with a patient, it is best to always present a dominant, "one-up" position.

2. If a patient successfully follows a suggestion, it is helpful to congratulate her.

3. Joining in is not an especially effective strategy for calming a hysterical person.

4. Asking a patient if he will follow your instructions is one way to achieve rapport.

5. Rapport with the second-in responder will occur automatically if the patient has rapport with the first-in responder.

EXERCISE

Write an introductory script you would feel comfortable using at a medical emergency. Practice it out loud until it feels natural.

What we nurture in ourselves will grow.
—Goethe

4 | Expectation

When a patient has expectations of things to come, he tends to make them happen. This chapter presents strategies for building positive expectations in the patient.

THE NEED TO SET THE STAGE

Emergency patients will follow simple directives quickly from someone they trust. The spontaneous state of consciousness that occurs during threatening times makes them hypersuggestible. Sometimes, however, more profound objectives like stopping bleeding or internally cooling a deep second-degree burn injury, require that you build expectations in the patient first. Such expectations set the stage for the acceptance of images that could influence the autonomic functions of the body.

BUILDING POSITIVE EXPECTATIONS IN THE PATIENT

The following communication strategies can be used to move a patient toward accepting beneficial suggestions that may initially be too unbelievable to accept. Note that one or more of these strategies may be used effectively in less than a minute and will not significantly delay your giving the desired directive.

Use Minor Successes to Achieve Major Ones

A basic principle of motivation is that success breeds success. When we are able to achieve one objective, we are more likely to attempt another. It is therefore wise to start out with relatively easy goals and to work up to more difficult ones.

Similarly, when patients act upon suggestions, they become less likely to oppose future ones. Each time a patient successfully follows a directive, expectation is built up for implementing the next one. Therefore, if time permits, it is best to start with easier ones and to work up to more dramatic ones. Easy directives include such things as asking a patient to tell you her name, to hold something for you, to cough or take a deep breath, and so on. After such directions are followed, be sure to congratulate the patient by saying "Good," or "Thank you," so as to frame the response as a minor success.

Give Assurance of a Hopeful Future

The most important thing you can do to build expectations is to give assurance that the patient's future is hopeful. This can be accomplished with both direct statements and indirect statements.

Direct Assurances
With direct assurances, care must be taken to avoid being unrealistic. Sentences such as "Everything is going to be fine," or "There is

nothing to worry about," will not be effective. The following examples of direct assurances are more likely to work:

- The worst is over.
- I'm an EMT and I'm going to help you.
- You're going to be OK.
- Things are being made ready for you at the hospital.
- The ambulance is on its way to bring you to the hospital, where the doctors will have you fixed up soon.
- By tomorrow this will just be something for you to talk about.

Indirect Assurances

Indirect assurances, when properly presented, can be the most effective way to reassure the patient. Indirect assurances are statements that imply that the patient will recover from the injury or illness. The following examples can easily be modified to fit the unique circumstances of each incident:

- I've found that many patients are able to _____ after I give them _____.
- When you get out of the hospital, I'd like for you to stop by the firehouse and say hello.
- It will be helpful when you are better if you try to avoid _____.
- Are you taking a vacation this or next year? Where are you going?
- I have a friend who had the same thing happen to him last year. He still has _____ (describing a *minor* symptom that would likely result from the injury or illness after initial recovery, only if needed for realism), but otherwise he made a 100 percent recovery.
- When you get well, I'd appreciate it if you would send me the address of the place you bought that (some interesting item owned or worn by the patient that might have value to you).

Thus, any indirect implication that patients will recover and be able to accomplish the requests you present will give them hope and increase their susceptibility to directives that will help them survive and recover.

Make Suggestions Contingent Upon a Physical Occurrence that Will Definitely Happen

With the contingency strategy, the desired objective is described in such a way as to make it seem contingent on something else you are going to do. This is done simply by stating the thing you are going to do or that the patient is going to experience and then suggesting that the patient will also notice some desired objective. The statement should be made in such a way as to matter-of-factly link the two objectives together—that is, to make them contingent upon one another.

This strategy can be used with a wide variety of medical interventions, from putting on a bandage or elevating the patient's feet to giving medication or administering IVs. In the following examples, a feeling of relaxation is made contingent on the releasing of a blood pressure cuff. (Contingencies work best when there is some obvious association between the two.)

> Now, I'm going to take your blood pressure. As the cuff deflates, notice how much easier your breathing becomes and how relaxed your muscles begin to feel. Good!

In a sense, the placebo effect is a contingency strategy. Confidently stating what an intervention will do will increase the effectiveness of the intervention. Here are some other examples of contingency strategy.

- This bandage will help stop the bleeding.

- This pill will improve your circulation.

- This position will make you more comfortable.

- If you take a full, deep breath right now, you'll notice that your heart rate will slow down considerably.

Offer Two Alternatives, Both Leading to a Desired Objective

If you ask a patient, "Would you be more comfortable with your arm at your side or across your lap?" he is not likely to present a third alternative. When the patient chooses by gesture, silent agreement, or verbal answer, he has accepted a degree of comfort in spite of his predicament. You can increase the focus on this comfort by saying, "Good. Just allow that feeling of comfort to spread through your arm and shoulders." But even without such follow-up, the patient's comfort level will have increased enough to build hopeful expectations for more suggestions from you.

The double-bind strategy thus provides the patient with an illusory freedom of choice between two possibilities, neither of which is really acknowledged as desired by him, but may actually be helpful to his welfare. Perhaps the simplest example of this, away from the emergency scene, is when children are reluctant about going to bed. If they are told they must go to bed by 8:00 P.M., they tend to fight against the order. If, however, they are asked whether they want to go to bed at 7:45 P.M. or 8:00 P.M., the majority will select the latter time of their own free will.

A simple double bind is to say, "Let's find out how much comfort this procedure will give you." The tacit implication is that it *will* give the patient comfort; the question is just how much.

Similarly, saying, "You might be surprised to find that you will feel more comfortable," the patient may challenge the statement by not being surprised to find comfort—or indeed to feel surprised at being comfortable.

The combinations of double binds at the emergency scene are limitless (legs up or down, strap tight or loose, blanket on or off), but make sure that both alternatives are appropriate for the medical treatment intended. For example, do not ask a patient who needs to be put in the shock position if she would be more comfortable sitting up or lying down.

Although numerous objectives besides comfort can also be used with the double-bind strategy, suggesting that a patient be more comfortable is preferable to phrases such as "less pain," "more oxygen," "less nervous," and so on. More will be discussed about this in Chapter 10, "Managing Pain."

If the patient does not answer a double-bind question, this sets up an opening for dropping the suggestion of *your* choice into her subconscious. Research has shown that, when someone is confronted with double-bind choices that are not negative, a disequilibrium momentarily occurs. With emergency patients, this imbalance increases receptivity for a *suggested* choice. Thus, after asking a double-bind question, if the patient hesitates without a reply, simply say, "I think you'll be more comfortable with your hand at your side."

Double binds can also build positive expectations when presented with future alternatives. For example, telling a patient who fears there will be no tomorrow that he will either feel hungry or a little nauseous in the morning, will tend to change his view. (This particular statement would be used only if neither event would be harmful, as the patient will most likely be one or the other if he indeed survives the immediate crisis.) Similarly, double binds can be set up with words like *expectedly* or *unexpectedly* or with phrases like "I don't know *which night* you will sleep the sounder," "if not now," "in a few minutes," and so on.

Guide the Patient's Images Elsewhere

Hopeful expectations build each time an emergency patient perceives a moment of relative comfort. The human mind can be programmed to ignore pain and sources of shock if directed to concern itself with times and places where pain and fear did not exist. If the patient can talk, this technique can sometimes be implemented by simply getting the patient to talk about work, hobbies, or family.

If talking does not seem appropriate, or when the patient cannot talk, you can guide her images elsewhere by asking her to imagine being in a far-off place. A smooth way to use this approach is to simply state, with a little levity, "I'll bet you can imagine someplace you'd rather be than here." Then, while administering medical treatment, ask what her favorite place is. In most cases, the patient will tell you. At that point, matter-of-factly suggest that she go ahead and go to that place in her mind's eye. Tell the patient that she only needs to come back when you or another paramedic speak to her. When the patient sees herself, even if briefly, in that place, she will be more calm and reassured. This will in turn increase the patient's positive expectations and inclination to follow your subsequent suggestions or directives. (More detailed description regarding images will be presented in later chapters.)

Utilize Ideomotor Response

One way to build the patient's positive expectations is to request for him to answer yes or no to questions by signaling with his fingers. This can be phrased as follows:

> For a few moments I want you to answer some yes or no questions for me by simply raising your index finger if the answer is yes [point to the patient's index finger and touch it] and the middle finger if it's no [point to and touch the middle finger]. If you don't know the answer or don't want to answer, just raise your thumb. [It's not necessary to touch the thumb.] You don't have to make very much of an effort to raise a finger, just a slight movement is sufficient. In fact, you might be surprised to notice the fingers will seem to answer the questions automatically.

At this point, you should begin to ask the patient appropriate yes or no questions. Depending on the state of treatment, this might include questions pertaining to medical history, the cause of the problem, positions of comfort, and so on. If verbal communication is preferred for these types of questions, you can use ideomotor signals when you begin a summary survey to locate specific areas of discomfort or injury. For example, "When I touch a place on your body, let me know with your fingers if you have discomfort there. Use the yes finger if you do feel discomfort, the no finger if you don't."

The reason ideomotor responses tend to build positive expectations is that they do seem extraordinary to the patient, as though the health care provider has tapped a powerful resource. Small motor neurons are activated in the appropriate finger when the patient begins to think of the answer. This results in movement that ranges from a slight twitch to a complete raising of the finger. Polygraphs utilize this effect in a similar way.

The paramedic should watch the fingers closely after asking the question. Even if a very slight movement of the finger occurs, congratulate the patient on the response. The patient herself will have noticed the movement, but it will seem to her as though it happened automatically, without effort. (In some cases the answers themselves may be more truthful than the patient would have wanted to answer. For example, if you asked, "Would you be more comfortable if your mother waits in the next room?" the individual consciously may not have wanted to hurt the mother's feelings and would not have expressed her truest feeling. The ideomotor signal, however, is more likely to react to the basic needs of the person. Since the patient realizes the priority for her own welfare, this also tends to build positive expectations.

Ideomotor signaling obviously also serves the function of two-way communication when it may be difficult for the patient to speak for one reason or another. This could be because of physical injuries, speech impairment, or even crowded conditions with many rescuers talking back and forth. In the latter instance, the ability to communicate with the primary paramedic simply and without effort can be of great comfort to a frightened individual. Of course, this requires that the paramedic give constant attention to the patient and continue to ask questions like, "Are you doing all right?" while rescue efforts are being made.

Another way to utilize ideomotor responses relates to patients who are being tended to while they are sitting upright, if they have the use of their arms and hands. Such patients may be given a pendulum device, such as a 2-inch section of string or chain with a weighted object on the end. (A paper clip will do.) Ask the patient to hold the end of the string between the finger and thumb with the weighted end hanging down. His elbow should be resting on the arm of a chair or on his knee. Have the person imagine the object moving back and forth in whatever direction he chooses. Although this may seem a bit far out, you can explain that this is simply an easy way for him to increase his comfort while you attend to his treatment or wait for the ambulance.

When the pendulum begins moving, most patients will be surprised, and the temporary distraction will have served to relieve their symptoms. If they appear surprised, tell them, "Many people are surprised when they see how they are able to effect a movement of the pendulum by merely visualizing it. It's nothing magic, it just shows how much more control you have over your body than you thought and how much more comfortable you can be." With this suggestion, positive expectations for the future will have increased. (Note: try the pendulum experiment yourself so you can have confidence in it.)

Eliminate Guilt and Anger

Both guilt and anger are emotions that result in negative expectations if they are not attended to properly. Such emotions are natural and can be beneficial if properly released but are poisonous if left unresolved. This is especially true for emergency patients who often feel guilt or anger in connection with their injury or illness. When we help a patient bring such feelings to a conscious level and then dismiss them, positive expectations are more likely to occur.

The best way to deal with a patient's anger is to change it into *constructive aggression*. Aggression, in its truest sense, simply means forceful action. This does not necessarily imply physical force, but instead the power of energy directed toward an objective. Such energy is natural to humans and should not be restrained. If the injured patient of an automobile accident is angry at the person who ran her off the road and is allowing the anger to build inside, then this emotion will impede her survival and healing mechanism *significantly*. Even if the patient attempts to ventilate the anger by verbal complaints like, "That SOB, he shouldn't have been in my lane!" the emotion remains stuck. Emotions are meant to move us toward constructive action. For example, if we feel fear, we have taken a positive action based on our interpretation of that fear; and then we move forward. Ill health only occurs if we remain focused on the fear.

In the case above, the driver who was run off the road feels out of control with her anger because her verbal self-communication has labeled the incident something that "shouldn't" have happened. "I know you're feeling very angry at the person who ran you off the road (joining-in strategy), but until we find out why he or she made such a mistake, let's take that energy and use it to get better."

Most individuals have enough of a sense of humor to appreciate such a reframing at the conscious level (though sense of humor varies a great deal from one person to the next). At the subconscious level, the reframe from "shouldn't have happened" to "should have happened" often allows the patient to move on without the anger resulting from being out of control.

Of course, this is only one example of ways to change anger into constructive aggression in the patient. The patient's manifestation of anger, the specific circumstances, and your own creativity and insight will mold the dialogue to fit each case. When the emergency patient's anger subsides or is transformed with the guidance of a rescuer, negative expectations are replaced with positive ones.

A similar approach is necessary for addressing feelings of guilt. Guilt, like anger, impedes the body's optimal healing and supports negative expectations of the future. As anger can be turned into constructive aggression, guilt can be turned into a creative mechanism for personal growth. In fact, guilt is an unnatural form of compassion. If someone feels guilt for having accidentally injured someone else, the paramedic can simply commend the feeling as evidence of natural compassion. When guilt is thus reframed, the patient is able to use the new perspective to learn from and grow with.

When emergency patients feel guilty for factors that may have contributed to their situation, they tend to view the pain and suffering as punishment. By giving an end point to the punishment, pain and suffering can be reduced. The following is an example:

Are you feeling guilty about having lit that cigarette in front of the gasoline pump? Well, listen, we all make mistakes. Besides, don't you think that what has happened to you up to this point has been sufficient punishment? OK, so go ahead and let that go now, and let's concentrate on getting better.

Incite Laughter Whenever Possible

Laughter, like crying, is a catharsis. It releases tension, pain, and stress. When laughing, it is difficult to be afraid. Laughter increases tissue oxygenation, disrupts muscular tension, distracts one from pain, and lowers blood pressure (after initially raising it). Laughter also decreases negative expectation and stimulates hope.

Although laughter may seem inappropriate to everyone involved at the emergency scene, if handled properly, it is a desired objective to get the patient to laugh at the pain, predicament, or embarrassment. If rapport between prehospital care provider and patient is high and some aspect of the situation is mutually laughable, a patient could be encouraged to laugh (depending on the nature of the medical problem) as another alternative for achieving the benefits of positive expectation.

In fact, a "laughable" rationale for laughing need not be a prerequisite. Like words, laughing symbolizes its own meaning within the cells of the body. When we laugh, our bodies respond positively. They do not care whether or not there was anything funny to laugh at. With this in mind, a confident rescuer could incite the patient to laugh at a predicament (again, only if the action did not complicate injuries or treatment), and it would significantly improve rate of recovery. Of course, be cautious that sufficient tact is used so the patient does not feel that the situation is not being taken seriously.

Propose the Use of Hypnosis

Most lay people have acquired definite expectations regarding the word, *hypnosis*. Few understand it for what it really is, but most have a notion of its power. In spite of the many misconceptions that a patient may harbor regarding hypnosis, the mention of it by a prehospital care provider, especially a professional paramedic or physician, may offer special expectations. In fact, if a patient indicates a willingness to use hypnosis to alleviate her symptoms, subsequent directives from the rescuer can be very effective. It is not necessary for the rescuer to induce a hypnotic state, since such a state of consciousness most likely already exists.

The proposal can be phrased something like this: "Are you familiar with the use of hypnosis in helping to alleviate symptoms similar to yours? Would you like me to show you how to use it? It can be very effective."

Unless the patient is obviously negative about the suggestion to use hypnosis, the rescuer can continue by using a simple hypnotic "ritual" followed by the desired directive. The ritual need be no more than telling the patient, "OK, I want you to take a deep, relaxing breath. Good. Now, when I count to three, just allow your eyes to close and begin to notice how much more comfortable you are beginning to feel."

At this point, a specific directive, phrased according to the guidelines presented in the next chapter, can be given. The expectations associated with the word *hypnosis*, combined with the serious need for help of any kind perceived by the patient, make this an effective strategy in many cases.

Since many of the techniques and strategies for effective communication presented in this book are similar to those used in clinical hypnotherapy, it may be useful to present a brief review of what hypnosis is and what it is not.

Hypnosis has been used and well publicized in the medical profession for almost two hundred years. In 1956 the AMA approved of it officially. Although it is often thought of as being a tool confined to psychosomatic medicine, it has been extensively used for surgical preparation and recovery. Dentists use hypnosis to control bleeding when operating on hemophiliacs. Many expectant mothers use hypnosis for painfree labor.

Unfortunately, the mystery behind the power of the mind has encouraged actors, writers, magicians, frauds, and religious leaders to convey the idea of hypnosis inaccurately. This, combined with a skepticism of things we do not understand, has added to the confusion about it.

In formal hypnosis, a client makes an agreement with the hypnotist to willingly suspend certain beliefs and allow himself to accept other beliefs for the moment. The language of the hypnotist helps the client's conscious mind to intensely focus so as to cut out other stimuli. This intensity of concentration cuts down barriers and allows the hypnotist's message to enter directly into the unconscious. Here, processes just beginning to be understood by science are acted upon.

In other words, hypnosis is the acquiescence of that alternative state of consciousness (often referred to as the unconscious mind) to a conscious belief. In formal hypnosis, the belief is put forth by a hypnotist. In everyday life, beliefs are put forth by mothers, fathers, teachers, advertisers, and ourselves. Some of them take hold when we naturally enter into the alternative state of consciousness. During emergency crisis, new beliefs are put forth by authority figures surrounding the frightened patient who is probably already in a state of spontaneous hypnosis. In all instances, the beliefs can influence the physical, mental, and biological functions of the person who has accepted them.

Before the use of the word *hypnosis* at the emergency scene, the state laws relating to the use of hypnosis should be reviewed. Although the laws are changing, a few states may still allow only licensed physicians to use hypnosis per se. In fact, if the receptive state emergency patients enter into can be called hypnosis, it would seem that first responders have no choice but to enter into a hypnotic relationship with them.

EXERCISES

1. What do minor successes have to do with building expectations?
2. Give an example of a way to offer a patient an indirect hopeful assurance.
3. Write a sentence that uses future alternatives in a double-bind strategy.
4. Why do ideomotor responses tend to build hopeful expectations?
5. In your own words, define hypnosis.

II | Suggestions and Directives

Words are the most potent drug that mankind uses.
—Rudyard Kipling

5 | General Directives

This chapter begins teaching specific guidelines for directing patients so that they may be able to tap optimal coping abilities.

When a first responder projects confidence, establishes positive rapport with the patient, and encourages hopeful expectations for the future in the patient, she has accomplished much. This alone will go a long way to activate the patient's survival and healing capabilities. When combined with appropriate medical care, this may be all that is needed to assure optimal treatment outcome.

In many cases, however, more specific directives or suggestions are required to tap all of the patient's biological resources. Limiting beliefs, fears, and/or memories may prevent the body from doing what it has the potential to do. A properly worded directive can bring about a specific objective, like a reduction in blood pressure, a decrease in inflammation, or a cessation of bleeding that would otherwise be dependent *only* on outside intervention (such as medication, ice packs, and pressure points). When properly formulated, such directives instantly create new beliefs that overcome the limiting fears and memories, thus allowing the body to express its full recuperative power.

Although directives for control of autonomic nervous system functions can be given to the emergency patient at any time, they are most effective after positive expectations have been developed. They may be given directly or indirectly as the following examples illustrate.

> Direct: You will be fine. This surgery has been successful with many patients.
>
> Indirect: You know, many patients wake up quite hungry from this kind of surgery and ask for unusual things to eat. If you have any unusual food preferences, let me know and I'll pass it on to your nurse.

or

> Direct: Stop that bleeding now!
>
> Indirect: When your arm stops bleeding in just a few moments, I'd like you to hold this cold pack on your knee.

Although both kinds of directives can be effective, it is the author's experience that indirect approaches meet with the most success. An exception is when signs of altered consciousness are very obvious. Remember, it can be presumed that all emergency patients are in an alternative state of consciousness that makes them hypersuggestible. Some, however, will be more deeply focused than others. With these patients, direct suggestions are very effective. Some obvious signs of this deep state of unconscious activity include

relaxed facial muscles

catalepsy

lacrimation

smooth facial muscles

When giving a patient directives that are intended to produce specific changes, it is, of course, helpful to know what those changes should be. For example, would it benefit the patient if his blood pressure lowered? Should blood vessels at a particular location dilate or constrict? Should a patient be encouraged to vomit or not? Is it best for a specific muscle to tighten or relax? Is an increase in body sugar called for? Would a patient benefit from antihistamine action? Is cooling or warming needed? Is more oxygen needed, or less? And so on. How accurately the rescuer answers such questions depends upon the level of his first aid-medical skills. If the specific biological, psychological, or physiological needs of the patient are unknown, directives can be more generally oriented toward the patient's getting better.

In most instances, nontechnical general directives that encourage remedial images for getting better are all that are necessary. (The advantage of technical knowledge lies in the increased opportunities for developing images.) When such hopeful, helpful directives are offered, the "window of the body" seems to be able to create the needed response. Similarly, this window also tends to protect the body from well-intended errors of judgment *as long as the mistaken directives were positive in nature.*

For example, if a rescuer directs a patient to dilate or widen blood vessels around the brain to make a headache patient more comfortable, but in fact the problem requires a constriction of blood vessels, research indicates that the hidden observer in the patient's mind accepts the general intent of the directive, but modifies the image to fit the more accurate response. On the other hand, if a negative, pessimistic, or frightening directive is phrased, experience shows that the hidden observer is less efficient in its ability to interpret the optimal response. (The following chapters will help ensure that proper phrasing of directives is accomplished.) For example, if the rescuer says, "I don't know if we will make it to the hospital in time, you'd better get your blood pressure down," the chances are that the blood pressure will not drop. *In any case, positive, hopeful communication, even when technically incorrect, is less hazardous than the incorrect administration of medications, IVs, oxygen, CPR, ice, and so on.*

EXERCISES

1. What is the hidden observer?

2. Give examples of direct and indirect suggestions or directives.

6 | Images

This chapter introduces seven guidelines to help assure that your words evoke positive images in the patient's unconscious mind.

CREATION OF LIFE-SAVING IMAGES

The goal of directives given to the emergency patient is to stimulate images that program healing processes. If the emergency is heat exhaustion, images that relate to cool mists, refreshing cool water, comfortable ocean breezes, or *whatever images the patient associates with becoming cool* can be encouraged. If the emergency involves a lacerated organ, imagery might relate to skillful carpenters entering into the bloodstream, finding the organ, and patching it. This image could be the rescuer's creative idea, or the rescuer may ask the patient to relate what she thinks of when thinking of something getting repaired. In the latter case, if the patient answers a carpenter, then the rescuer can build on this image. *It must be remembered that the images are symbolic.* A carpenter patching something that is broken is a symbolic image that the patient can utilize to direct actual healing processes.

The power images have over our actions and normal mode of thinking is depicted by the following illustration: If a 4-inch plank is set on the ground and you are asked to walk the length of it, you would probably have no problem assuming you had the physical skill to do so. However, if it is placed between the roofs of two tall buildings and you are asked to walk across it, the *imagined* possibility of falling would have more influence over your balance than even a high monetary incentive to accomplish the task.

It is the creative part of guiding images that the first responder may find the most challenging. This is only because of inhibitions about such childlike communication at the emergency scene. Our culture has tended to discourage, rather than encourage, such imaginative discourse. Fantasy has been relegated to the nonproductive side of our existence. The irony is that most of the billions of brain cells we possess relate not to logical, linear thinking, but to imaginative thinking. This inhibition to describe such imaginary ideas will quickly disappear as the effectiveness of such communication becomes more and more obvious.

DEVELOPING HEALING IMAGES

The following guidelines, combined with a willingness to express your own natural creative imagination, are all that is necessary to help a patient develop healing images.

Utilize All Five Senses when Developing Imagery

When we think of imagery, we often think only of visual imagery. However, imagery can also involve the senses of touch, taste, hearing, and smell. In fact, when several senses are combined, images tend to be more vivid. For example, a person might be more apt to respond to an image of being relaxed by the ocean if he could feel the warm sand, hear the ocean waves crashing into the shore, smell the seaweed and kelp, taste the salty mist, and see the blue skies and green, frothy ocean.

Make Language Understandable to the Patient

The less left brain activity required to comprehend directives, the more image-producing activity will be available. It is therefore important to speak clearly, slowly, and in terms the patient can easily understand without having to think about meanings. By avoiding any ambiguity in your language, you will help the patient create images quickly.

For similar reasons, it is also helpful to make use of the patient's language. Of course, this means speaking in a person's native language when possible. Even if a patient is bilingual, it is an advantage to speak in the individual's first language. This is because, during early childhood, this language was associated with much imagination. Also, it was the language that authority figures like mother and father spoke, and it may facilitate rapport.

Making use of a patient's language also means using slang or regional or occupational phrasing if the paramedic is familiar with it. When this is done, however, care should be taken to do so without parody or seeming to put the patient down.

Use the Patient's Own Experiences

Imagery works best when it is the patient's images, not the rescuer's. A place that is relaxing to one person is not necessarily going to be relaxing to someone else. For example, a paramedic may ask the patient to imagine lying in the sun on the beach because that is *her* idea of being relaxed. The patient, however, may have had a bad experience in such an environment that was anything but relaxing. It is thus always better to ask the patient what would be a relaxing place for her. Then you can direct her to go there and encourage associated images to form.

The author has asked hundreds of emergency patients to describe a happy, comfortable place with the following wording: "I'll bet you can imagine someplace you'd rather be than here right now." Then, after a few moments of working on the patient, ask, "What place did you imagine when you thought of a place you'd rather be?" Almost without exception, patients in all levels of distress have identified a unique spot.

Be Descriptive

Since the emergency patient is not going to feel much like talking, it is up to you to embellish an image with descriptive details so as to color it and make it potent. The following experiment may illustrate the importance of descriptive adjectives when stimulating imagery. Read it through, then set the book aside and try it.

> While resting comfortably in your chair or bed, allow your arm to rest at your side. Now imagine that your arm is raising upwards. Do this for a few moments.
>
> Remembering what sensations you had, if any, now refocus on your arm again. This time, imagine that a bunch of brightly colored helium balloons—red ones, blue ones, green ones, and many of your favorite colors—are all tied by a string to your wrist. See them uplifting in the clear, blue sky. Notice how they rise when a brisk summer breeze blows them. You might also imagine them becoming bigger with each breath you take, causing your hand and arm to lift ever higher.

In most instances, the latter image will have been more effective in causing the arm to lift than the first one. The more colorful the description, the more vivid the image. Thus, with a patient of cold exposure, you would not just have that person imagine a warm place, you would have him imagine the following: being in the warm sand, feeling the hot sun rays beating down, or, being wrapped in a cozy, soft blanket in front of a big stone fireplace, with the orange flame reflecting heat all over his body and the aroma of a burning oak filling his nostrils. Tell the patient to imagine hearing the crackling and sparkling of the burning embers and his body becoming warmer and more comfortable.

Use Emotional, Exciting Words

Besides being descriptive, your words should have an emotional, exciting intonation and emphasis. It is not known exactly why this increases the imagery potential, but it is thought that it relates to early childhood imagination experiences. During this time, parents and other adults typically speak to children with a tone of emotional excitement in an effort to encourage positive images. For instance, "What a *big* boy! You lifted that *great big brown* box *all* by yourself," or "What a *beautiful* picture you have drawn. Just look at the *pretty red* flowers." Apparently, such language during times of stress tends to stimulate latent imagery cells and also tends to encourage increased receptivity to parental-type guidance and assistance.

Thus, instead of saying, "Your heart is beginning to beat more regularly now," say "*All* the fibers of your heart muscle are beginning to work *together* now as a *team, pumping fresh, oxygenated blood* to *all* of the cells in your body." The tone of excitement and emotion in your voice will intensify appropriate images and will also seem to validate them. (If you doubt the power of emotional rhetoric, tune in to a TV evangelist some Sunday and see how he is able to motivate people to contribute to his organization!)

Use Only Positive Phrasing

One of the most important things to remember when speaking to emergency patients is to phrase your statements in the positive. Words like *not* or *won't* do not form images in the mind; therefore, images are produced by the object of the sentence that uses them. Directives that contain negations should therefore always be re-phrased.

Wrong way: You're not dizzy any more.
Right way: You're feeling clear-headed.

Wrong way: In a few moments you won't feel like crying.
Right way: In a few moments you will feel more relieved.

Wrong way: Don't breathe so fast.
Right way: Breathe slower.

Wrong way: You are not going to die.
Right way: You are going to live.

The following example demonstrates this point: A golfer wants to hit the ball down the fairway in between two ponds. If she says to herself, Don't hit the ball in the pond, or I will not hit the ball in the pond, what happens? The image-producing quality of the words *pond, hit,* and *ball* overshadows the word *not*. As a result, subtle body messages will tend to hit the ball into the pond as imagined. If, however, the golfer says to herself, I will hit the ball *down the fairway,* she is more likely to do so.

In addition to negative statements, words with negative connotation should be avoided. The most common such word used in communication with emergency patients is *pain*. When a paramedic or a physician asks the patient if he has pain or where the pain is, he has offered the image of pain to the patient. Since any phrase that uses the word *pain* is still going to nurture the image, it should almost always be replaced with the word *discomfort*.

Wrong: Tell me where you feel pain.
Right: Tell me where you feel the most discomfort.

By using the word *discomfort* instead of *pain*, you are now able to form a directive to reduce the pain without using the word—for example, "Notice how much *more comfortable* you are becoming." A good way to work with pain is to ask the patient to describe his discomfort on a scale of 1 to 100. Then, using the strategies that have been discussed and the examples in Chapter 10, "Managing Pain," ask the patient to see himself at improving levels.

Remember, if the patient can hear what you are saying, it is important to substitute the word *discomfort* for the word *pain* when reporting the injury to the hospital or to personnel taking over the treatment.

Attach Triggers to Images When Called For

A *trigger* is a symbolic action that reintroduces a helpful image automatically. For example, you might tell a patient that whenever she touches her finger and thumb together, the feeling of comfort will quickly and automatically return. Shrugging the shoulders, smiling, taking a deep breath, blinking the eyes, and so on can serve as a trigger.

Triggers give the emergency patient a sense of security and control. When being transported to the hospital and away from your confident directives, a patient can use the trigger whenever needed to keep your directives working if and when other reactions temporarily block them.

Situation:
A patient with a crushed hand has been treated by the rescuer and is responding well to suggestions for pain management. The ambulance has arrived, and the patient is about to be lifted onto the stretcher. The rescuer speaks to the man:

Louis, if later on you need to regain the feeling of relative comfort that you are feeling now, all you need to do is take a deep breath, exhale, and touch your finger and thumb together. As soon as you do, that feeling of comfort will come flooding back automatically. Go ahead and do that now. Take a deep breath, exhale, and touch your finger and thumb together. Notice how much more comfortable that makes you, even now. Good.

TRUE OR FALSE?

1. When developing imagery, only the visual sense should be targeted.

2. A day at the beach would be a relaxing image for everyone.

3. "You are not dizzy now," is a proper directive.

4. A trigger helps a patient bring back a useful image when needed.

7 | Believability

*Since the patient is aware at both the conscious and
unconscious level, directives must appear relatively
believable. This chapter presents rules that will help the
patient keep this perspective while still stretching the
limits of his imagination.*

BELIEVABLE DIRECTIVES

Much has already been said about the importance of credibility. Images follow beliefs. During crisis, victims tend to believe the directives of a confident authority figure with whom they have rapport. They believe in the possibility of the images to which they are guided.

If directives are given incorrectly, however, belief in them may be challenged by the patient both at a conscious level and at an unconscious level. Incorrect directives that disrupt believability usually result from violating one or more of the three basic rules described in the following sections.

Directives Should Be Relatively Accurate

Relatively accurate means being as honest and as accurate as possible, *without* validating the patient's fears. This relative accuracy accomplishes several objectives. First, when the rescuer can be honest, he can remain confident. Remember that an emergency patient's intense focus on his problem keeps that person highly tuned in to those persons within his focus of attention. When we are consciously deceptive, we signal subtle lapses in confidence.

Second, the more accurate the basis of a medical treatment description, the more believable it will seem to the patient. This does not necessarily mean being technical in language. For example, if you are encouraging someone to manifest images that will enhance the immune system, you do not have to talk about T cells and theta brain states. It would be sufficiently accurate to speak of immune cells banding together to rid the body of infection, while other cells relax.

Third, being honest and fairly accurate in your communication with the patient will keep the patient believing in you, thus maintaining rapport.

There is often a delicate line between telling the patient what is going on at the emergency scene or answering questions about the patient's condition (or the condition of his friends or relatives) and holding back information so as not to increase fears about the future. The following illustrations will exemplify ways to avoid crossing the line.

Situation:
An automobile accident with multiple casualties has occurred. The rescuer is treating the adult driver who has possible spinal injuries and broken ribs. This patient's young child, age ten, is dead. The rescuer knows this. The injured driver does not.

Patient: Where's my little boy? How is he? Oh my God, is he all right? Please, someone tell me!

Rescuer: I know how worried you are about your son. There's a paramedic working with him right now, and he's an excellent paramedic. I know he is taking good care of him. The best thing *you* can do for him is to help me do everything we can for you, too. You can begin by keeping your head still while I put on this brace. While we're doing this, I want you to . . .

In this delicate situation, the rescuer manages to be accurate and honest without revealing information that could be detrimental to the patient's survival potential.

Situation:
A right-handed thirty-four-year-old male has maimed his right hand in machinery at work. Future use of hand is unlikely. Patient appears in control and has looked at his hands.

Patient [speaks after treatment for pain and bleeding has been administered]: Will I ever be able to use my hand again?

Rescuer: I truthfully don't know. I do know that they are able to do incredible things with reconstructive surgery and that injuries almost always look much worse than they are. You'll probably be surprised to see how much you'll be able to do with that hand after a while.

This illustration shows that the amount of information you reveal to the patient is in part determined by how much the patient already knows. Believability is risked if you contradict what the patient knows for sure. At the same time, however, care must be taken not to validate the patient's negative beliefs.

Another way to increase believability is to start with a relatively easy directive and work up to more profound ones. A basic principle in psychology that relates to suggestibility is that suggestions that are acted upon create less opposition to subsequent ones.

Use the Progressive Form of the Present Tense when Phrasing Directives

Although a direct imperative like, "Stop your bleeding *now*," can be effective, directives are more likely to be effective if they are phrased so as to give the patient more leeway to accept the appropriate images—for example, "Your arm is already beginning to feel numb," or "Notice that your arm is beginning to feel numb." This type of phrasing suggests that the patient should become aware of something that is already happening but she may not have noticed it yet. With this approach, there is less chance that the victim will resist a directive. There is also less chance that rapport will be lost because something you said did not happen right away. Instead, the patient has time to work up to the image.

Forming directives in the present progressive also helps prevent the patient from trying too hard to comply. Another basic tenet of psychology is the law of reversed effect. This says that the harder you try to do something, the more likely it is you will fail. A directive like "Lower your body temperature, now," may increase activity in the left brain where willful determination is initiated. However, unless strong, positive success images also exist, willful determination involved in trying to do something somehow reinforces images that relate to the difficulty or inability to be successful. For instance, the harder you try not to blush, the more likely it is you will blush, and so on. Present progressive directives seem to *assume* success, rather than demand it.

Make Directives Relative to the Patient, Not the Environment

Directives are believable or possible when they relate to potential changes in the patient, rather than those things outside her. This is because, in fact, the patient's images can only influence her own mind-body complex, not external objects, persons, or events.* The following examples illustrate this point:

> Wrong way: Notice how much cooler it *is* outside.
> Right way: Notice how much cooler *your body* is becoming.
>
> Wrong way: Imagine how quickly the help will come.
> Right way: Help is on its way. You might be surprised to see how fast the time will go by until they arrive.

---

*There are hints of evidence that an individual's images can affect external realities. Theories relating to this have been presented in the arenas of philosophy and, more recently, in physics. Whether such psychic energy actually exists is a question that may someday be answered when the disciplines of psychology, philosophy, medicine, neurophysiology, and other physical science join forces. Until then, we might assume that, at least indirectly, what we imagine can influence the world outside us. (See Chapter 19, "Saving the Planet.")

Wrong way: The ride to the hospital will be quiet and relaxing. Right way: Notice that all the sounds you hear, including the siren and traffic noises, will *add* to your experience of comfort and relaxation.

As with most rules, this one has an exception. It is all right to direct an image that relates to what a medication will do as opposed to how the body will react to the medication, though a directive could be formed either way. As with the placebo effect, belief in the external power of the substance triggers internal images. Ultimately, however, it is the belief in what the drug will do for the body that can influence its success or failure. (Refer back to experiment with ipecac in Chapter 1, "Credibility.")

An interesting example of this ability was demonstrated by author and psychic Edgar Cayce. A physician administered injections to the unconscious Cayce, not knowing that Cayce was in control of his recovery from an apparent illness. Rather than suffering any ill effect from the injected drug, Cayce whispered to a friend to tell his body to "reject the drugs." With this directive, the medication actually withdrew from its initial systemic path into bumps just under the surface of the skin.

EXERCISE

Give five directives for five different emergency situations, using the progressive form of the present tense.

Words cannot be remote from reality when they create reality.
—John Cowper Powys

8 | Literal Interpretation

During the first hour or so, a person in trauma has a tendency to interpret statements quite literally. This chapter illustrates two important ways to avoid giving the patient the wrong idea.

THE LITERAL INTERPRETATION OF LANGUAGE

For directives to achieve the desired results, the paramedic must remember that his words will be interpreted quite literally by the patient. Images are stimulated by their initial perception of meanings. Analytical brain functions that might otherwise be able to put the word or words into context are not operating during stress. Recalling Dr. Wright's description in Chapter 1 of what happens to the frightened emergency patient, we see that "the person's usual critical responsiveness to the environment has been altered so that (information is) subject to a *literal translation* and can either aggravate or support the life systems" usually considered to be under control of the autonomic nervous system.

FORMULATING DIRECTIVES

The following sections give you guidelines that will help you formulate messages from which the patient can make appropriate literal translations.

Avoid Phrases with More than One Meaning

Generally, rescuers and paramedics can avoid literal misinterpretation by keeping conversation simple and patient-directed. When slang or conversational phrases that could be misinterpreted by the patient are avoided, whether to the patient or between rescuers, the chances of such problems are significantly diminished. The old joke common around fire departments depicts this point well. (It probably actually happened once upon a time!) It goes something like this: "Did you hear about the accident patient who was pinned inside his car? He didn't have any injuries, but he died of a heart attack when he heard the fireman call for the 'Hurst'!"

Fire fighters usually get this joke because they use the word *Hurst* to refer to a hydraulic tool also called the "jaws of life," which is used to open crushed-in doors. The tool is manufactured by a company called Hurst, Inc. Obviously, the subject of the story thought that the call for a "hearse" meant the end of the line.

This joke may or may not be an extreme example. Either way, such words uttered in jest may become fixed in the patient's mind and cause untold harm (as mentioned in Chapter 1, "Credibility"). Every effort should therefore be made to avoid phrases that may have more than one meaning. Putting someone to sleep may mean something quite different to the patient who just put his German Shepherd to sleep than to the anesthetist who was merely referring to a general anesthetic.

With some effort, it is not too difficult to choose sentences carefully when speaking directly to the patient. It is more difficult to control them when speaking to others. Remember that the patient's entire focus of attention is related to his predicament. As a result, anything that is said before a patient is construed as pertaining to him. If the patient overhears someone say, "He's not going to make it this year," a statement referring to the paramedic's son's prospects for making the football team, the patient assumes the sentence is about himself. He assumes that no one could be talking about football when someone's life is on the line. Even seemingly innocuous phrases like, "He's out to lunch," could be damaging to the patient. A paramedic may simply be telling her dispatcher that one of the paramedics is on a lunch break. The patient may interpret the phrase to mean his condition is much worse than he imagined. Taking a few moments to think before speaking with this point in mind is an important rule for effective communication with the emergency patient.

Affirm Activity, Not Ability

A second guideline that relates to the patient's literal interpretation of communication is to make sure directives describe *activity*, not *ability*. For example, telling a patient, "Notice that you have the ability to stop your bleeding," is not as effective as saying, "Notice that your bleeding is beginning to stop." If the patient accepts the image of the first directive, she will indeed believe she has the ability to stop bleeding, but the mind will not direct the body to do it.

Similarly, the use of the word *try* should be avoided because of the literal translation. If you direct a patient to try and breathe regularly or to try to be more relaxed, the patient will literally *try*. Only when your directive says, "You are breathing more regularly," (direct) or "You are beginning to breathe more regularly" (present-progressive), will the desired objective occur.

Simple biofeedback exercises demonstrate the ineffectiveness of "trying," even with people who are not in stress. When hooked up to biofeedback monitors, participants who are not trained in imagery, self-hypnosis, or relaxation responses increase anxiety profiles when they are asked to try to relax.

In psychology, a strategy referred to as *paradoxical intention* is often used to elicit change. This involves asking a patient to *try* hard to do the negative behavior. For instance, a patient whose hands sweated whenever he met a new person (and tried to keep his hands from sweating) was told to try his best to sweat more than ever on the next occasion. The results were that he did not sweat at all. Although the author has not used or has not seen this approach used with an emergency patient, it may be worthy of experimentation when dealing with relatively *minor* complaints. For example, if a patient was complaining about extreme itching all over her body, this strategy might be employed as follows:

> Patient: I can't stand it. I'm itching everywhere!
>
> Medic: I know how horrible it must feel, but I think I can help you. I want you to *try* as hard as you can to make your right arm itch more than your left. Go ahead and focus your attention on your right arm and really try.

Theoretically, the law of reversed effect could work. If the right arm itch were reduced, the technique could be used elsewhere. As mentioned, since the author has no research supporting this approach with emergency patients, experimentation should only be done with minor problems. In more serious situations, the risk of not including the word *try* and just focusing on an image of the objective might exist. Thus, saying, Try to bleed, could present the wrong response.

EXERCISE

Give three examples of words and phrases that could have more than one meaning.

Enthusiasm is one of the most powerful engines of success. When you do a thing, do it with all your might. Put your whole soul into it. Stamp it with your own personality. Be active, be energetic, be enthusiastic and faithful, and you will accomplish your object. Nothing great was ever achieved without enthusiasm.
—Ralph Waldo Emerson

9 | Enthusiasm

This chapter describes how the right amount of enthusiasm can be a significant factor in patient communication.

THE ROLE OF ENTHUSIASM

The last letter of our CREDIBLE mnemonic is a reminder of the importance of enthusiasm when you are involved in assisting an emergency patient. Enthusiasm underlies success in projecting confidence, gaining rapport, building positive expectations, and giving successful directives. If the strategies that have been discussed are not working for you, increase your enthusiasm and note the difference.

To get an idea of how a statement, with and without enthusiasm, compares, try this. First say, "The worst is over. Things are being made ready for you at the hospital," without any sense of enthusiasm, energy, conviction, or sincerity. Just say it as though you were tired, bored, and unconcerned. Notice how it would feel if you were a patient.

Next, repeat the two sentences, this time with enthusiasm. Be convincing and caring. Be alive and put your own personality and style into it. Now, imagine how the patient would respond.

What exactly is enthusiasm, how do you get it, and how can it benefit communication with the emergency patient? The word itself comes from the Greek word *enthousiasmos* meaning "inspired." Webster defines it as "ardent interest." Synonyms include the following: *vigor, energy, animation, drive, esprit de corps, potency, spirit, vitality,* and *devotion*.

Note that all of these qualities enhance characteristics of leadership. They are things that make a patient want to follow your directives with equal enthusiasm. If you are without enthusiasm at the emergency scene and an enthusiastic bystander is talking nearby, the *patient may focus on the bystander's words and not yours*. Since the bystander has not learned the principles of effective communication, she may very well say something that could significantly hinder the recovery of the patient.

Your level of enthusiasm, especially while at an emergency scene, is determined by your emotional reactions to people and events. These reactions, no matter how internalized they may seem to you, emit energies that are picked up by the emergency patient. Any reaction that negates your energy, your devotion, your esprit de corps, your inspiration, or your potency robs you of enthusiasm.

BALANCE IN ENTHUSIASM

As with all aspects of optimal health, balance with regard to enthusiasm is important. Too much enthusiasm can make communication as ineffective as too little enthusiasm. Like too little enthusiasm, too much is also related to your emotional reactions to things. Ultimately, control of your emotional reactions starts with self-awareness.

To make more sense of this important aspect of communication with the emergency patient, let us go through an example of how to develop and project appropriate enthusiasm.

Increase Your Self-Awareness

Start with self-awareness. Using the following psychological traits, score yourself on how much or how little of each trait you now possess. Think of these in relation to how you behave at the emergency scene.

desire

assertiveness

sensitivity

tension control

confidence

personal accountability

self-discipline

Let us take the trait of assertiveness, for example. Assertiveness is feeling that you can affect the treatment outcome of a patient. Give yourself a low score if you are easily intimidated by a patient, a situation, or other rescuers. Give yourself a high score if you are not. Also take a low score if you are too assertive to the point of being insensitive. Overassertiveness can be a greater problem than under-assertiveness because it manifests itself as insensitivity. (Picture the paramedic who arrives at the scene, ignores the first responders, and goes right to the patient without asking questions, then proceeds to cut the patient's clothes off while giving orders to everyone in an aggressive tone.) If your score is near the middle, your emotional reactions to things that relate to your assertiveness are probably not going to affect your enthusiasm negatively.

The next step is to note the emotional reaction that relates to this trait when some event or person brings it into play. Is it fear, anger, jealousy, anxiety, worry, insecurity, embarrassment, and so on? Imagine yourself at an emergency scene and see an event that relates to this personality trait and the reactive emotion. After you have done this, substitute a more appropriate emotional response and mentally rehearse it with the same emergency scene. With practice, the reactive emotion will become reprogrammed and your self-rating for the trait will change.

Stay in the Present Moment

Whether or not you go to the trouble to work through the previous exercises, your level of enthusiasm will improve if you understand the connection between enthusiasm and serenity. This relationship is best described by the anonymous saying that is the motto of Alcoholics Anonymous:

> God, grant me the serenity to accept the things I cannot change,
> The courage to change the things I can,
> And the wisdom to know the difference.

In a sense, enthusiasm exists in its most perfect form when one is able to accomplish all three of these objectives. Furthermore, this is best accomplished if you can learn to concentrate fully on being in the present moment. This is true because the only way to be in the present is when you *instantly accept emotionally whatever happens at the emergency scene.* This point is well illustrated by the Zen story of a monk who was being chased by two tigers. He came to the edge of a cliff. He looked back—the tigers were almost upon him. Noticing a vine leading over the cliff, he quickly crawled over the edge and began to let himself down by the vine. Then, as he checked below, he saw two tigers waiting for him at the bottom of the cliff. He looked up and observed that two mice were gnawing away at the vine. Just then, he saw a beautiful strawberry within arm's reach. He picked it and enjoyed the best tasting strawberry in his whole life!

Notice that the monk fully responded to the physical danger in the most intelligent way. His emotional reactions did not relate to his past or future fears or concerns. By being in the present, the emotion that emerged was enthusiasm. This is what the emergency patient most requires.

If being in the present nurtures enthusiasm in the rescuer, would being in the present also be beneficial for the patient? Some evidence indicates the answer is yes. Although patients need positive expectations for a hopeful future to *replace* negative expectations, *once this is achieved,* the individuals do better when their thoughts remain in the now.

> Wrong: Go ahead and think about how nice it will be to be with your family later, and notice how much better you will feel.

Right (after negative worries for the future have been canceled): Notice what is going on around you. Let all the sounds become part of your experience of comfort.

One of the most effective approaches to building appropriate enthusiasm, for both rescuer and patient, is to reframe or redefine problems as being challenges. It is difficult to face problems with enthusiasm, but challenges can always be met enthusiastically.

Wrong: I know this is a terrible problem for you, but we are doing our best to help you with it.

Right: This may be one of the greatest challenges you will ever have to face, and it offers a great opportunity for you to show how well your inner resources can respond.

Put yourself in the patient's place and hear both statements. Which one is most likely to promote life-embracing enthusiasm?

TRUE OR FALSE?

1. Directives should stimulate only images that involve visual sensations.

2. The following directive would be appropriate: "In a few moments, you won't feel any pain."

3. If one directive is followed, a second directive is less likely to be successful.

4. The future tense should always be used when phrasing directives.

5. The following directive would be appropriate: "You now have the ability to lower your blood pressure."

EXERCISE

Score yourself on the traits listed on page 75.

III | Specialized Directives

The determination of an heroic effort will be
remembered long after the pain is forgotten!
—Unknown

10 | Managing Pain

This chapter discusses appropriate language to use with
people complaining of severe pain.

PAIN TOLERANCE

The emergency patient's tolerance for pain is influenced by a class of biochemicals called endorphins. These are substances very similar to morphine that are produced by the brain. Endorphins block pain by filling certain neuron receptors so that other chemicals that carry pain messages cannot come in.

Exactly what causes the production of endorphins and what regulates the amount of endorphins is not understood. What is known is that emotions, attitudes, thoughts, and external verbal and nonverbal communication can significantly influence the production of endorphins. This explains why seriously wounded soldiers who know that their injury will allow them to return home for the duration of the war often report only mild discomfort. It also may explain the agonizing suffering of phantom limb pain even when the patient's stump is anesthetized.

Since methods of pain control are relatively easy to measure experimentally, numerous studies have been done in this area. In most cases, the opiatelike substances produced by the brain proved to be more potent than the administration of pain-killing drugs. For example, a National Institute of Health study, published in Volume 296 of the *Annals of the New York Academy of Sciences* compared hypnosis, acupuncture, morphine, valium, aspirin, and placebos in the management of experimentally induced pain. Tolerance of pain was measured by timed exposure to an ice-cold surface and to ischemic pain resulting from a blood pressure cuff set at 300 mmHg . With both types of pain, the greatest protection was afforded by hypnotic suggestion of analgesia. (The second most effective was 10 milligrams I.M. of morphine per 70 kilograms body weight.)

Thus, the experience of pain appears to be largely subjective. You may recall emergency patients with relatively minor injuries expressing extreme pain and others with more serious injuries expressing little. You may also remember the emergency patient who did not complain of pain until you started talking. In these instances, the painful *sensation* of the injury did not become the painful experience of suffering until communication triggered an inappropriate subjective thought about the injury.

If pain is not being expressed by the patient on a conscious level, either verbally or nonverbally (indicated by grimacing, muscular tension, etc.), then there is no pain experience. Do not create a pain experience with inferences that pain must exist. The easiest way to do this is to simply avoid using the word *pain* at all in your communication. If you need to ask the patient questions about her pain so as to help you diagnose her problem, phrase your sentences more in line with the following example.

> *Situation:*
> *The rescuer arrives at the scene of an emergency involving a forty-three-year-old male who has fallen from a 14-foot ladder. He is on his back—alert and conscious—and is exhibiting no signs of pain. After checking for bleeding, and while putting on a C-collar, the rescuer begins his secondary survey to determine where the patient is injured.*

Wrong: Mr. Bloom, before we can help you we need to know where you are *hurting* or where you are feeling the most *pain*.

Right: Mr. Bloom, so we can know where to begin, it would help us if you could describe exactly what place on your body needs attention.

> *Similarly, during the secondary survey with a patient who is not expressing pain, avoid use of the words* hurt *and* pain, *which are likely to start subjective responses that will increase the pain experience. Instead, use the word* discomfort.

Wrong: Tell me if I touch a place where you feel pain. (Or, tell me if I find a place that hurts.)

Right: Tell me if I touch a spot where there is some discomfort.

ALLEVIATING PAIN

If you are called to an emergency where the person is in obvious pain, there are a variety of directives you may choose from to alleviate the patient's perception of pain, thereby encouraging the production of endorphins. One or more of the following techniques can be used without interrupting standard care.

Give a Suggestion to End the Guilt-Punishment Cycle

Many emergency patients who are suffering from acute pain feel some degree of guilt about the accident that caused the pain. In most instances they know some act of negligence, ignorance, or omission on their part contributed to the accident. When this happens, the pain serves as a just punishment in their mind for this sense of guilt.

If your statements to the patient can bring this idea of guilt to the surface and can then show that enough punishment has already occurred, the resulting relief will diminish the perception of pain.

Situation:
A twenty-four-year-old woman was involved in a car accident—she has injuries and is crying in pain. The rescuer speaks to her.

Mary, I may be wrong, but I sense that you are blaming yourself a little for this. Even if there was something you could have done to avoid this, don't you think that what has happened is punishment enough? Good, now let's get on with fixing you up!

A similar emotion is fear or anger. ("That really scared you, didn't it? You don't think that guy really meant to run you off the road. He probably swerved to miss a deer.") Forgiveness is the treatment of anger.

Give a Directive to Increase the Patient's Sense of Control

The more helpless an emergency patient feels, the more likely he will suffer from pain. The expression of suffering is a way of calling out for help. Whenever you can involve the patient in the treatment of the injury, this sense of helplessness can be reduced. However, when you give a directive that gives the patient some control over the pain itself, a significant improvement can be gained.

An effective directive for giving the patient direct control over the pain can be patterned after the following.

Situation:
A twenty-eight-year-old female was hiking and has badly twisted her ankle. She is experiencing extreme discomfort.

Susan, the distress you are experiencing is your body's way of telling you that something is wrong. But the signal doesn't have to be as loud as it is for it to reach you. In fact, you can control the volume of the signal while at the same time telling us when we are helping and when we're not. Just imagine that there are colored electrical wires running from your ankle to a light bulb in your brain. Between your ankle and the light in your brain is a dimmer switch that dims or brightens the light. When messages from your ankle head up to the light to signal your discomfort, you can intervene to control the intensity of the signal. Just to see how easily this works, go ahead and *begin to dim* the light a little now. Good. Now you maintain control with the dimmer to whatever level you need to let us know what is happening.

Direct the Patient to Understand a More Important Priority than the Injury

In some medical emergencies, there is an urgent need to remove the patient from the scene as quickly as possible. When this occurs, the patient's perception of pain can be changed by getting her to recognize the more important threat. For example, a boxer is likely to ignore pain until the fight is over.

> *Situation:*
> *A hiker has broken her leg on a steep, remote mountain trail. Access by helicopter is impossible, and the cold night is approaching. Paramedics have to maneuver the gurney down over rocks and ravines. The task will be almost impossible after dark.*
>
> Joanne, I know how terribly uncomfortable this is for you. However, I want you to help us out as best you can by remaining as still and as quiet as possible. If we don't get you off this mountain before dark, we're all going to be in trouble.

You should be cautioned that this type of directive should only be used with a patient in pain whose injury itself is not life-threatening. Even in such a case, a positive outcome should be implied, although it is made contingent on their cooperating with the rescuers.

Guide the Patient Toward Healing, Comfortable Images

Directives that help the patient visualize ideas or things that would reduce pain are very effective. What these may be is limited only by your (or the patient's) imagination.

> *Situation:*
> *A sixteen-year-old male was riding a horse alongside another horse that kicked him in the shin and fractured his tibia. The boy does not have a good tolerance for pain and continues to complain vehemently. He describes the pain as being sharp and piercing, as though a knife were being jabbed into the bone. Good rapport exists between him and the paramedic, however, and positive expectations have been encouraged.*

Danny, as I wrap this cotton bandage around your leg and the cardboard splint, I want you to close your eyes for a moment and visualize the cotton being so thick and so matted that nothing could pierce through it. When you see that image, next see a sharp knife jabbing at the area but it can't get through to your leg. You feel the pressure as it jabs into the cotton, but you are much more able to stand this amount of discomfort. Good.

When you reach your tolerance level for this dull discomfort, see the knife being withdrawn from the cotton and notice the feeling of relief. Good.

Now, Danny, on your way to the hospital you can repeat this process whenever you need to. Just imagine more and more cotton being wrapped around your leg and notice the decrease in discomfort and the increase in comfort. The extra energy you have can now be used to speed up the healing. And remember, don't be mad at that old horse anymore—he wasn't aiming at you.

A second example of the use of guided imagery to reduce the pain experience is seen in the case of an acute abdomen patient. Acute abdomen problems such as appendicitis, peptic ulcer, kidney infection, and so on can cause severe localized pain. Treatment in the field is limited to anticipation of shock and efforts to transport to the hospital as quickly as possible. Since the patient's knowledge of interior anatomy is usually less than what is known about external anatomy, there is often more confusion and fear about what is going on. Guided imagery can replace fearful, counterproductive images with images that can help the healing process.

Situation:
A forty-seven-year-old male with a history of peptic ulcers is complaining of extreme pain in the lower right quadrant of the abdomen. During transport the paramedic utilizes guided imagery with the patient. He speaks matter-of-factly about the use of guided imagery.

Mr. Vaughn, are you familiar with how the use of mental imagery can redirect certain biochemical processes in the body? Well, it's very effective. We'll be at the hospital in about ten minutes and in that time we can do quite a bit to not only make you more comfortable, but also to enhance the healing process and to help your body respond wonderfully to the doctor's treatment later on.

What I'd like you to do is close your eyes, and as you do, notice the immediate increase in comfort. Now, just allow that feeling of increased comfort to increase even more. As it does, notice that you *are beginning* to relax the muscles around your abdomen a little more and that this also increases the sense of comfort. Good.

Now I want you to imagine that a crew of special miniature workers are going down into your stomach to fix the problems that are causing you discomfort. See them going down to fix a sort of protective seal that is in need of repair and that is allowing stomach acids to get into the stomach lining. *What kind of tools do you think they could use to fix that seal?* [In most instances the patient will offer an idea, such as a special glue, and so on. If not, suggest your own creative imagery.]

Good. Now just begin to see this miniature crew working very efficiently as they caulk around the broken seal with the soft, jellylike sealant. And as they do, notice that less stomach acid is allowed to get into the damaged area. Good, it's beginning to work. Just keep on with the work. Soon we'll be at the hospital and whatever treatments you get will serve as help to the miniature workers!

Give Directives that Shift the Patient's Attention to Another Time and Place

Directives can be used to shift the patient's orientation to a time or place when pain was not experienced. By drawing attention to a happy memory or thought, the mind is not able to pay as close attention to the pain messages.

Situation:
A thirty-year-old male was using a blowtorch to cut through an empty oil drum to make a barbecue. Fumes remaining in the drum were ignited and the resultant explosion lacerated and burned the man seriously. During treatment, the first responder attempts to reorient to a different time and place.

I'll bet you can imagine some place you'd rather be than here. As a matter of fact, go ahead and do that now while we get you bandaged up. Think of your favorite place. When you are there in your mind's eye, look around and notice all the things there are to notice. Listen to the sounds. Feel the good feelings. There might even be a special aroma you can smell. When you are really experiencing that place, let me know by raising your index finger. Good.

Induce a Relaxation Response

During an emergency, the nervous system accelerates heart rate, respiration, and blood supply to the muscles. Even after real danger is over, the continuation of these responses tends to keep the patient feeling a sense of danger and pain from the injury. If a relaxation response can be attained, these reactions become reversed. When heart rate, muscle tension, and circulation are relaxed, the patient often feels freedom from pain even in the middle of the emergency.

Since the idea of relaxation during an emergency is likely to be seen as being unrealistic to the patient, the relaxation response is best achieved when it is associated with a specific realistic reason—for example, having the patient relax so that an accurate reading can be taken with the blood pressure cuff; or a man with angina pain is likely to understand that by slowing his heart rate he can better fill his coronary arteries. Once a realistic association is made, directives for relaxation are likely to be accepted. Note that direct suggestion for relaxation can be tied in with directives described in the preceding section.

Situation:
A twenty-two-year-old male hiker dislocated his left shoulder during a slip and fall on the trail. He is ten miles from the nearest access point to emergency help. One of his companions runs for help. The second stays with him. Trained in these procedures of communication, he proceeds to help his friend:

Pete, while we are waiting for John to get help, I want to tell you what I know that can make you more comfortable. The terrible discomfort you are feeling is happening because your arm and shoulder muscles are tight and are straining the tendons and ligaments that have been stretched. If you relax the entire arm and shoulder, those relaxed muscles would ease the strain. [In some cases the muscles will relax so much the shoulder can easily be relocated, even though this is not recommended for paramedics to attempt.]

Now, when I count to three, I want you to take a deep breath and then let it all the way out. As you exhale, notice the muscles in your arm and shoulder relaxing. Then, they will continue to relax more with each exhalation.

Give the Patient a Way to Change the Intensity of Pain

When the pain experience cannot be removed, it is relatively easy to help the patient modify it. An easy way to do this is by using a pain scale, having the patient locate where on the scale the pain is, then encouraging her to go lower on the scale.

Situation:
A twenty-eight-year-old female injured her knee during a marathon run. Swelling and pain are severe.

Susan, in a moment I want you to describe the level of *discomfort* in your knee on a scale of 1 to 10. Let the number 10 be the most discomfort you can imagine, like a knife jabbing in your knee or a red hot iron, and let the number 1 be a mild pressure like someone just touching you with their finger. *You may be surprised* to see how easily you can change the level, upwards or downwards, from where you are now.

For example, tell me where you are now with your knee on that scale. [The patient says 8 or 9.] OK, now, just for a moment, move it down and tell me where you moved it to. [The patient says 6 or 7.] Good. Would you be willing to move it back to 8 or 9 for just a moment? [Patient either agrees or prefers not to. If he does not want to, that is fine. If he does, it increases his sense of control, and he may next move it all the way down to 3 or 4.]

Give a Direct Suggestion for Comfort and Pain Relief

For extremely frightened emergency patients, direct suggestions can be quick and effective—for example, "The discomfort in your head is gone," or "When I count to three, your head will feel clear and comfortable." The risk with such directives, however, is that they may not work. The patient may not be ready for them. When this happens, you lose a little rapport and you might even lose some self-confidence. Nonetheless, there will be times when such directives are appropriate.

Situation:
A forty-two-year-old female was pinned behind the wheel of her car with multiple injuries. Two other cars were involved in the accident and there are three injured people in each car. The female driver's chest is pushed hard against the steering wheel, and she is hysterically screaming about her pain. The rescuer and her part-

*ner are involved in assigning triage priorities while waiting for
more help. The woman's screaming is frightening other patients
on the scene and is preventing the rescuer from examining her
condition effectively. When speaking to hysterical patients, it is
often helpful to place a confident, firm, but gentle hand on a
shoulder and speak softly into their ear. Patients tend to better
concentrate on words that are whispered in their ears when in this
condition. The rescuer speaks to the woman.*

I know how much you are hurting and how scared and
maybe even angry you are, but the *worst is over now*. Soon
we'll have you and your friends out of here, but we need
your help. Will you help us? Good [whether or not patient
actually agrees]. Now, first you need to breathe easier.
When I count to three you'll notice how much easier and
more relaxed it will be for you to breathe. One, two, three.
Good.

Give a Directive for Glove Anesthesia

Another kind of directive that can be given to alleviate pain is called
glove anesthesia. This refers to a technique used in medical hypnosis to
prepare patients for surgery when chemical anesthesia is not desired.
Although it is a direct type of suggestion, it gives the patient a feeling
of control over her pain. When time permits, an emergency patient
can be taught how to use glove anesthesia to control her discomfort at
will.

Situation:
*A twenty-four-year-old male is a patient after a beating. He has
multiple contusions (bruises). He is conscious. Whenever paramedics try to move him, he resists and complains of pain. None of
the injuries appear to be life-threatening, and the rescuer has
managed to establish a positive rapport with him. The rescuer
decides to utilize glove anesthesia because it will give control back
to this patient.*

Arnold, I'm going to give you a powerful tool that you can
use *any way you choose to help yourself feel better*. In fact, you
can reduce the discomfort and increase the healing at any
particular place on your body where you need to. OK, just
look at your fingertips for a moment and notice how you
can make the tips of them numb as though they were all
sprayed with novocaine. Touch each fingertip with your

thumb and notice how the feeling is going away, as though you were touching the rubber fingers of a mannequin or a doll. Good. You can allow that *feeling of numbness* to spread up your fingers and into your hand until your entire hand begins to feel numb, or it may feel cold as though it were being dipped into ice water.

Now, whenever you are ready, you can use this hand to transfer this cool or numb feeling to any part of your body that would benefit. For example, go ahead and touch the bump on your forehead and notice how it also becomes cool or numb. Notice, too, how much more comfortable that feels.

Arnold, we are going to put you in the gurney now. Whenever you feel discomfort, just touch that part of your body where you need it the most.

PAIN MASKING

Pain serves a purpose. It is a warning that something is wrong. Once the warning is heeded, however, the pain becomes unnecessary. Emotional factors such as fear and other learned perceptions usually maintain pain and suffering until these things no longer serve a constructive purpose. However, to the degree that first responders and emergency physicians need to know what is wrong with the patient, it is not desirable for *all* of the patient's pain to go away.

The above directives will not usually cause all the pain to disappear. The patient will be more comfortable and may stop suffering, but they will still be able to communicate about the source of the pain. However, particularly responsive patients may mask over the pain completely. For this reason, each directive you give should include a suggestion for the patient to keep just enough discomfort at the injury site so that he can continue to tell you the effect of the treatment and so that he can tell the same to the doctor. This suggestion has the added benefit of giving control for the pain back to the patient.

EXERCISE

You have a patient complaining of severe pain in his fractured elbow. Describe exactly what you would say (and how you would say it) to help relieve the pain.

The blood also thinks inside a man, darkly and ponderously. It thinks in desires and revulsions, and it sometimes makes strange conclusions.
— D. H. Lawrence

11 | Stopping Bleeding

This chapter deals with the patient's ability to follow directives to stop her own bleeding.

*T*he variable amount of bleeding from similar wounds in different emergency patients has been of interest to many professional first responders. One person's laceration may bleed intensely. Another's may not bleed at all. Often, a patient does not start bleeding from an injury until after the paramedics arrive and start talking.

The ability of some individuals to voluntarily control bleeding is well documented. Numerous surgical procedures involving hypnotic suggestion or acupuncture have been accomplished with unusually small amounts of bleeding. One study, described in the BBC film, *Can Your Mind Control Your Body?* showed a major reduction in bleeding during dental surgery with two hundred hemophiliacs. Without hypnotic suggestion, the hemophiliacs required from five to thirty-five transfusions of blood. With hypnotic suggestion they required from two to three.

It is not known precisely how thoughts or directives physiologically decrease hemorrhage. It seems to relate to constriction of blood vessels and coagulation of blood as well as to some other basic biochemical changes. David Cheek, M.D., an obstetrician and a pioneer in the use of medical hypnosis, has speculated that the sudden cessation of arteriolar and venous bleeding is due to high outpouring of epinephrine followed by the relaxation of muscles surrounding the injury. Epinephrine does increase coagulation speed of blood. But normally rebound fibrinolytic activity causes secondary bleeding. Perhaps confident directives to relax and stop bleeding inhibit internal messages to send fibrinolysins to the injured area so that the initial response to the epinephrine is maintained. Whatever the processes involved, directives to stop bleeding can be very effective at the emergency scene. The following case studies illustrate the kind of phrasing you may want to use.

Situation:
A thirty-four-year-old woman was thrown from a vehicle in a multiple car accident and is bleeding from a small artery in the lip and from a deep laceration in the scalp by the time help arrives. After taking a moment to appraise the situation and gain self-confidence, the paramedic puts his thumb on the woman's forehead to get her attention and says, "Listen to me. You are OK. Stop that bleeding now." The woman stops her bleeding, and the paramedic goes to look at another patient. A bystander yells out, "You'd better get those people away from the car before it blows up—there's gasoline leaking!" At that point, the first patient starts crying and her bleeding begins again. The paramedic quiets the bystanders, assures everyone that there is going to be no

explosion and returns to the patient, again placing his thumb on her forehead. "Listen to me. The worst is over. Now stop that bleeding. You did it before and you can do it again." Again, the woman's bleeding stops and arriving paramedics begin direct pressure bandaging and stabilization procedures.

Situation:

A twenty-two-year-old male bicyclist not wearing a helmet suffered a scalp laceration when his bicycle spun out coming down a steep hill. Upon arrival, the fire fighters find the patient alert and completely oriented. He is badly shaken, however, and frightened enough to be in an alternative state of consciousness as evidenced by his hypersuggestible, smooth facial expression and fixed eye staring. Bleeding has stopped, but the hair is matted with blood and the wound is filled with road dirt and debris.

Bill, you can start and stop your own bleeding by simply concentrating on turning it on or off. We need to clean some of the debris out of your wound, and it would help us if you would go ahead and allow it to bleed again just for a moment. Go ahead and do that now. Good, that helps.

While the paramedic cleans out the debris with a sterilized 4-by-4-inch pad, the patient begins oozing blood that helps with the process. After about ten seconds the wound is prepared for bandaging. Direct pressure bandaging is applied, and Bill is asked to stop the bleeding again:

OK, Bill, we've got the wound clean and we can bandage it now. When I count to three, I want you to stop the bleeding again.

It is interesting to note that there seems to be a reduction in infection of cuts when an individual uses mental processes to control bleeding. Dr. Esdaile found this to be true with his surgery in India, as has Jack Schwarz, who has demonstrated this ability numerous times around the world. Schwarz "sterilizes" 6-inch needles by rubbing them on the floor with his shoes before sticking them through his biceps to show his ability to stop pain and bleeding.

Situation:

A five-year-old female lacerated her arm while playing with a razor blade. Her mother finds her crying several moments after it happened. Venous bleeding is significant. The mother maintains a calm, confident manner and tone of voice and, having been trained in these communicative procedures, manages to calm her daughter and encourages her to stop the bleeding.

Oh my gosh! Oh, honey, you cut yourself with that sharp razor. It hurts, doesn't it? Sure it does! And look at all that blood. That's really good, healthy, strong red blood you've got. And, you know, you've bled just enough to make sure that your cut is clean. So now you can go on and stop the bleeding while you hold this washcloth against your cut. OK?

The child holds the cloth against her wound, stops crying, and stops bleeding.

Situation:
A fifty-four-year-old male with a history of stomach ulcers has vomited blood. His pulse is thready, his skin is clammy, and his eyes are dull. The patient states that he is thirsty and that he is afraid he is going to die. While the two arriving paramedics administer oxygen, place the patient in the shock position, and wait for the ambulance, one of them has managed to gain rapport and build expectations for a positive future using several strate-gies outlined in the previous chapters. He is now ready to give a directive to get the patient to stop the internal bleeding.

Mr. Edwards, as you know, your stomach is probably bleeding again. You can stop that bleeding yourself, and I'm going to tell you how. I want you to imagine, just imagine, that you have sent a crew of workers down into your stomach to patch up the places where it is bleeding. Will you do that? Just imagine them *any way you choose,* but see how quickly and efficiently they are able to patch up your stomach and stop the bleeding. Good. That image is already working. Your blood pressure is beginning to sta-bilize. Now, I want you to continue with those images all the way to the hospital.

Since standard field treatments are minimal for internal bleed-ing, whether from a bleeding ulcer, a broken rib, a closed fracture, or a bad bruise, this approach might result in saving lives.

EXERCISES

1. What strategy has the mother employed to help her child stop bleeding in the situation described on page 96?

2. Using the case of the fifty-four-year-old male with a bleeding ulcer (page 96), create your own directive using descriptive metaphors to create images that could help stop the bleeding.

12 | Cardiovascular Emergencies

Your ability to calm and reassure the heart patient can prevent secondary attacks and can do much to stabilize vital signs. This chapter discusses how to effectively speak to such a patient.

SHOCK

Thoughts have a significant influence on our cardiovascular systems. States of anxiety can raise blood pressures and heart rates. Relaxation can lower them. Furthermore, people can learn to control these functions voluntarily, though they are usually considered to be involuntary nervous system responses. Yoga masters have demonstrated the ability to drastically raise or lower their pulse and blood pressure, as have students training with biofeedback equipment. Similarly, meditation classes have been extremely effective in helping hypertensive patients manage their blood pressure without drugs.

During medical emergencies, the action of the heart and blood vessels is affected by a variety of conditions. Such conditions can cause the patient's nervous system to dilate or contract the size of the arteries and veins, thus raising or lowering blood pressure. If the blood pressure is too high, vessels can rupture. If too low, vital organs may be seriously damaged and life threatening shock may occur. Since so many conditions, from anxiety and blood loss to infection and bee stings, can lead to shock, treating for shock is always a first aid priority for most medical emergencies.

Preventing or treating shock has generally meant repositioning the patient so blood can return to the heart more easily (preventing further loss of blood and body heat), giving oxygen, and applying pneumatic counterpressure garments when available (and if the first responder is qualified). However, none of these procedures take full advantage of the tremendous capability of the patient's own autonomic nervous system. Since the adaptive ability of the nervous system is often compromised by misdirected or overactive thoughts, new directives can help restore equilibrium in the same way that falling down can restore normal perfusion in the person who has fainted (psychogenic shock).

It is relatively easy to give patients directives for raising or lowering heart rate and blood pressure, once confidence, rapport, and expectations have been gained. It should be noted that individuals can control either function independent of the other. In other words, a patient can lower her heart rate without changing blood pressure or vice versa.

Situation:
A fifty-three-year-old female is showing signs and symptoms of shock, including a weak and rapid pulse rate of 120 and a low blood pressure of 100/60. Her skin is clammy and pale. She is conscious, and she tells the rescuer she has had severe nausea and diarrhea for several days.

100

The rescuer talks to the patient on the way to the hospital.

Martha, you've lost lots of fluid and it has been difficult for your heart to pump oxygenated blood to all the parts of your body. Just imagine a garden hose with a small volume of water running through it. Notice how slowly the water drips out of the end. But if you narrow the size of the opening, the water comes out faster. Your body can adjust the size of your blood vessels to compensate for the loss of water. Go ahead now and allow your body to make those adjustments so that oxygenated blood can be carried to all the parts of your body that need it, especially your brain, your heart, your lungs, and your kidneys. Just begin to feel how these organs are right now being given adequate amounts of oxygen rich blood.

Research has shown that individuals can learn to direct increases in blood flow to specific locations in the body. For example, Elmer and Alice Green of the Menninger Foundation have taught patients to vasodilate vessels in the hand so that hand temperatures have increased by as much as twenty-five degrees Fahrenheit. By asking emergency patients who may be going into shock to concentrate on blood flowing to those vital organs that cannot lack perfusion for very long, cardiovascular responses may enhance survivability until more technical medical procedures can be applied at the hospital.

ACUTE MYOCARDIAL INFARCTION (HEART ATTACK)

The mind-body connection seems particularly obvious when referring to injury to the heart muscle. Even the traditional poetic metaphor, as in "You have broken my heart," points to this connection. Theories that suggest that some personality types are more susceptible to acute myocardial infarction (AMI), or heart attacks, also infer that the health of the heart is linked to mental processes. And, there is little doubt that emotional stress and anxiety can significantly influence heart function and blood pressure.

Once a heart attack has occurred, it is likely that mental considerations become even more influential on physiological responses. Some studies show that many deaths result, not from the initial heart attack, but from secondary attacks that relate to anxiety about the first one. The extremely frightening nature of having a heart attack makes the patients extremely responsive to proper communication from attending rescuers. Since the nervous system remains capable of coordinating heart fibers, increasing or decreasing heart rate, and reducing inflammation in heart tissue, directives that create appropriate nervous system image-responses can be lifesaving.

> *Situation:*
> *A forty-six-year-old male with a history of mild hypertension has suffered a heart attack. When the responder arrives on the scene, the patient is conscious and describes a substernal pain characterized as "squeezing" and radiating to his jaw and left arm. The pain has lasted for over an hour. Heart rate is 140.*

Mr. Davis, it appears that you have had a minor heart attack. I know how frightening the feeling you have now seems, but the worst is over. Your body is now trying to regain a homeostasis or balance, and if you do what I say, I can help you regain that status more quickly. Will you do as I say? [The patient acknowledges in the affirmative.] Good.

> *Up to this point the rescuer has projected confidence, given the patient positive expectations for the immediate future, and, through the direct contract strategy, gained positive rapport. Remember to speak calmly and professionally. One of the common aspects of acute myocardial infarction is a feeling of impending doom. As patient anxiety increases, so does the number of irregular heartbeats. If this is allowed to continue, the arrhythmia may produce disorganized ventricular activity followed by fibrillation and death.*
>
> *Although telling the patient that his body is now trying to regain homeostasis or balance may in itself be a sufficient indirect suggestion to regain a normal heart rhythm, at this point a more specific directive can be helpful.*

OK, Mr. Davis, I want you to concentrate on breathing in this fresh, pure oxygen from the mask and send it to your heart to help the uninjured muscle fibers carry on the efficient, organized work of pumping that oxygenated blood through your body. Now I really want you to imagine, in whatever way you choose, that those heart muscle fibers are regaining their composure and are beginning to work smoothly again. You might imagine a team leader down there directing the group of muscle fibers to work in an efficient, coordinated way, easily compensating the tissues that were injured. As you do this, notice that you are beginning to slow your heart rate down. Since the team is working so efficiently now, fewer beats are required to get the work done. Good. You're doing well.

CARDIAC ARREST

A large percentage of all individuals who suffer an AMI go into cardiac arrest. This means the heart has stopped beating altogether or is in a state of completely disorganized quivering, called fibrillation. The chance to save such a patient exists only if treatment can be administered within a short time, usually about three to four minutes. In many cases, immediate initiation of cardiopulmonary resuscitation (CPR) has been responsible for patient survival of cardiac arrest. CPR in itself, however, is comparatively inefficient, and success rates for reviving patients of cardiac arrest are not high. Perhaps if internal mental forces could be tapped during CPR, more effective results could be achieved.

Numerous anecdotal experiences indicate the validity of possibility. First of all, David Cheek and others have demonstrated that unconscious individuals continue to be aware of what they construe to be meaningful sounds. Dr. Dabney Ewin has reported responses in heart rate and blood pressure to verbal commands in surgical patients under general anesthesia. If the nervous system can be directed to regain normal heart rhythm in a conscious patient, it may be able to stop fibrillation or even restart heart beat during asystole.

An example of this may have occurred recently in an Oakland, California, emergency room. A young paramedic who had been a student of the material presented in this book brought a patient in cardiac arrest to the emergency room. He had been continuing CPR en route to the hospital, thus sustaining the patient's life artificially. The emergency room physician began working on the patient. At the same time, he confidently spoke to the paramedic:

"It looks like this fellow is going to be all right, doesn't it, paramedic." Overjoyed to find a physician that seemed knowledgeable about patient communication, the paramedic matter-of-factly replied, "Yes. It looks like he is going to make it." Just at that point, the electrocardiogram (EKG) tracings that had been showing a straight line jumped into a normal heart rhythm pattern.

When the paramedic told me the story, I asked him who the physician on duty was. It turned out to be Dr. Lee Balance, an experienced emergency room physician who was a speaker at the First International Conference on Emergency Hypnosis held in Mexico in 1984. Apparently, the communication strategy the doctor and the paramedic used was no accident.

Just as positive directives and hopeful statements can revitalize an injured heart, negative, anxious, or panic-filled words may stifle the most efficient application of CPR. Unfortunately, first responders doing CPR on an unconscious patient do not often appreciate the fact that they are treating an extremely frightened individual who can indeed respond to what is being said. Once a patient gives up hope, a broken heart becomes a literal description.

A case in point is described by Dr. Deepak Chopra in his new book, *Quantum Healing*. He describes an overstressed fire fighter who was suffering symptoms of heart problems. Numerous thorough examinations revealed a healthy heart and vascular system. Nonetheless, the fire fighter kept returning to Dr. Chopra complaining that he was having heart problems.

After a time, Dr. Chopra recommended a full-service connected retirement for the fire fighter, based on occupational mental stress. The retirement board rejected the retirement application. Several days later the fire fighter died from a massive heart attack.

Whether this case illustrates the powerful influence of negative expectations on the heart or was simply an example of an undetected heart problem, we will never know for sure, but Dr. Chopra's follow-up research made him conclude it was the former. Thoughts and images affect the functioning of our cardiovascular systems perhaps as much or more than any external intervention. It is a responsibility of the first responder to use the communication skills described in this book to attempt to direct those thoughts and images in a positive manner.

Situation:
A fifty-three-year-old male has suffered a heart attack. His wife is trained in CPR and, after determining the absence of a pulse, she begins CPR immediately after witnessing the cardiac arrest. The rescuer arrives within fifteen minutes to commence two-person CPR after determining the continued absence of a pulse. The following communication is spoken to the patient calmly and professionally during CPR without interrupting it.

Louis, my name is Don. I'm a fire fighter/EMT, and I'm here to help you. I know you can hear me, and I know you are very frightened. Your wife and I are helping you supply your body with oxygen until you can do it on your own. The ambulance is on its way and things are being made ready for you at the hospital. It's important for you to help us, Louis. You are doing OK, but we need you to take a breath on your own. OK, Louis, let's get your heart beating regularly again. You are going to be all right, but we need you to help us now.

Throughout the entire time CPR is being given, this kind of dialogue should continue. It should not stop until the patient is revived or until he is pronounced dead by a physician. I cannot emphasize the importance of this. As long as you are making an effort to revive the patient with your hands and oxygen bottle, you must continue with your communication efforts. I have personally talked to survivors of cardiac arrest with whom I used CPR. These individuals all stated that the personal, consistent, and confident communication somehow helped them stay in the fight.

STROKE

In the fourth edition of *Emergency Care and Transportation of the Sick and Injured*, the authors describe the prescribed treatment for stroke patients. This includes the following statement: "The single, most important aspect of the treatment for this patient is thoughtful, tender, loving care." They thus acknowledge the importance of a kind of communication that can reduce complications that result from anxiety and fear.

Since many stroke patients will not be able to speak to you at the emergency scene, you must look for signs that indicate that the patient is responding to your communication. Such signs could be as subtle as the blink of an eye. A better way to set up a communicative structure is to ask the patient to answer yes to questions by raising the index finger and no to questions by raising the second finger. Ask for the response on the unparalyzed side. The ideomotor reflex (described earlier in the text) will thus be activated and will serve three functions. First, it provides an immediate opportunity for two-way communication; second, it gives the stroke patient a sense of control, in spite of the debilitating nature of the injury; and third, it helps create a special rapport between you and the victim.

When a stroke occurs, an interruption of cerebral blood flow damages a portion of the brain. This impairs some biochemical or physiological function that was initiated at the site of injury. Although we know very little about the brain, we do know that the majority of brain cells are not activated regularly. We also know that certain portions of the brain can learn to take over functions usually controlled by other areas. For example, at New York University Medical Center, stroke patients were taught to regain motor activity using electromyographic feedback. These patients developed new internal sensory circuits from the brain to the affected motor neurons. As a result, normal functioning returned.

Because of the rapid learning potential emergency patients have while in states of spontaneous hypnotic consciousness, it is possible that your directives could cause a stroke patient to quickly regain control of some vital function at the emergency scene, while standard procedures are being implemented.

> *Situation:*
> *A sixty-eight-year-old female has difficulty with speech and partial paralysis on the left side of the body. While standard first aid procedures are being initiated, the rescuer is speaking calmly and confidently to the patient.*

> Mrs. Bradley, I know that you can hear me, and I know that you are very frightened about what has happened to you. You have had a blood vessel injury in your head that has temporarily immobilized some of your muscles. While your brain figures out how to compensate, we are going to help you by . . . [Describe interventions being used such as suction equipment, oxygen, bleed pressure, etc.] In a few minutes I'm going to show you how you can begin using the uninjured portions of your brain to assist your breathing and your swallow reflex. Right now I want you to just close your eyes and imagine being in some favorite resting place of yours. The ambulance is on its way, and things are being made ready for you at the hospital. Now, if you can understand what I am saying, I want you to indicate that by raising the index finger on your left hand. You don't have to raise it very much, just a little will do. Go ahead and do that now. [Patient responds.] Good. Now, go ahead to that special restful place while we put you on the gurney and get you ready for our drive to the hospital. Let me know by moving that finger when you are at that place in your mind's eye. [Again, patient responds.] Good.

> *At this point the rescuer can attempt to give a more profound directive that might allow the patient to regain control of some vital function, such as breathing regularly, that might be at risk for further complications or failure. The rescuer has built up expectations for it with the phrase, "while your brain figures out how to compensate."*

OK, Mrs. Bradley, your body is already beginning to heal from your stroke in its own way. The doctors are waiting for you at the hospital. Until we get there, however, there is much you can do to get other portions of your brain to help you control your breathing. It won't be easy because you have been doing it one way for a long time, but if you are willing, try, and I'm sure it will help. Are you willing to try? [Patient responds positively.] Good. Now, all I want you to do is to notice that you have different ways to signal your chest muscles to move and to signal your diaphragm to move. Experiment until you are able to take a little breath on your own.

If vital functions are not in jeopardy, the rescuer will probably not choose to direct the patient to learn how to activate a paralyzed muscle group at the emergency scene. This is best reserved for the physical therapist. However, if directives can help save the patient's life, this approach is certainly worth trying during the extra time that is available while waiting for the ambulance or during transport to the hospital.

Note that, for both heart attacks and strokes, it is often just as important to use effective communication with the patient's family as it is with the patient. For guidelines relating to this, see Chapter 17, "Psychological Crisis."

TRUE OR FALSE?

1. The inability to calm and reassure victims of heart attacks may be responsible for fatal, secondary heart attacks.

2. Speaking to an unconscious victim during CPR is a waste of time.

3. Patients can be directed to control such autonomic nervous system functions as pulse rate and blood pressure.

The wind that fills my sails propels, but I am
helmsman.
—George Meredith

13 | Burns and Environmental Emergencies

The inflammatory reaction to burns is especially
influenced by communication and thoughts that affect
the autonomic nervous system. This chapter discusses
how and gives examples of how to talk to a victim of a
burn or other environmental trauma.

BURNS

One of the most dramatic effects of the CREDIBLE mnemonics communication approach is with burn victims. The pain and fear associated with this kind of insult to body tissue create a tremendous inflammatory response by the autonomic nervous system. In the case of deep second-degree burns, this response often requires patients to go through months of painful surgery. With proper communication at the emergency scene, however, this inflammatory response, along with fever, pain, and blistering, can be drastically reduced. In many cases, patients suffering deep second-degree burns recover in one to two months without surgery, significant pain, or disfiguration.

The basis for the profound influence of suggestion or directives with burn victims has been illustrated in numerous clinical and field studies. For example, hypnotized individuals have created burn blisters after being told that a cold coin placed on the arm was extremely hot. Other subjects have been burned with lit cigarettes but did not develop a burn blister when suitable directives were given. (Several examples of such experiments are documented in the BBC film, *Can Your Mind Control Your Body?*)

The phenomenon of fire walking also illustrates the ability of the body to react to heat in such a way as to diminish pain and inflammation. Studies of fire walkers in Fiji and India indicate that a strong belief system is responsible. In India, fire walking is preceded by a three-week meditation ritual. In Fiji, fire walkers are told from birth that they have been given this special ability. In the United States, the author and others have successfully walked across 1,500-degree coals, barefoot, using hypnosis. In all cases, some image formed in the mind stopped that part of the burning that triggers the pain and inflammation response.

In a research project conducted by Gerald Kaplan, M.D., director of the acclaimed burn center at Alta Bates Hospital in Berkeley, California, it was demonstrated that hypnosis facilitated dramatic enhancement of burn wound healing when vasodilation to the burn site was suggested. In the project, burn patients were selected on the basis of having bilaterally equivalent burns on some portion of their right and left sides. Since only one side of the body was treated by hypnotically induced vasodilation, the patients served as their own experimental control. Four of the five patients demonstrated clearly accelerated healing on the treated side only. The fifth patient had rapid healing to both sides.

In the above study, directives for increasing blood flow to the injured site were given one or two days after the burn, while the patients were still in the hospital. Dr. Larry Moore, a clinical psychologist and hypnotherapist, hypnotized the patients with their permission, and suggestions (directives) were given while patients were in the hypnotic state of consciousness. It is important to note that two aspects of this procedure are *not* required at the initial emergency scene. First of all, as has been stated already, frightened and confused individuals in the throes of a medical emergency automatically enter into what can be called a hypnotic state of consciousness that makes them extremely receptive to properly worded directives when the CREDIBLE guidelines are followed. Formal hypnosis procedures are not necessary.

Second, and most important, effective directives for burns that are given within one or two hours after the initial injury call for vasoconstriction to the burn site, *not* vasodilation. This difference is similar to the standard treatment for a bruise or sprain, where cold is applied immediately after the injury and heat applied after a day or two. Dr. Dabney Ewin, a diplomate of both the American Board of Surgery and the American Board of Medical Hypnosis, has been reporting successful treatment of burn injuries since 1978 with confident directives that move the patient toward feelings of cool and comfort. Such feelings relate to images that lead to vasoconstriction.

Suggestions for constriction of blood vessels at the burn site, when given within one hour post burn, probably reduce the inflammatory process in several ways, since all inflammatory reaction is orchestrated via the autonomic nervous system. The sooner directives are given, the more effective the treatment. It is easier to influence the nervous system with directives before it begins sending messages on its own.

Although this apparently would not work for third-degree burns, where nerve endings have been entirely destroyed, it does work for all burns where nerve endings are still operating.

The photographs on the color insert illustrate the effectiveness of Dr. Ewin's treatment with an emergency patient who was burned by an acetylene torch when the hose broke. (Acetylene burns at three thousand degrees Celsius.) He gave the patient suggestions to keep the injury cool and comfortable until it healed. The communication took place within one hour post burn at the hospital emergency room. Dr. Ewin gave the suggestion while placing cool towels over the wound. There was no scrubbing of the wound. Although the towels had a temporary physiological cooling effect, they also enhanced the image capability for coolness in the patient.

The heat from the torch was sufficient to vaporize the patient's shirt and charcoal his skin. Nonetheless, no pain medication was necessary, and, at twenty-one hours, no swelling or edema existed. There was even wrinkling of the skin distal to the burn. The patient returned to work the next day! In just eight days, the charcoaled skin began peeling off and healthy skin was showing beneath it. In twelve days, the wound was healed with no scar tissue or permanent burn scar.

For many burn patients, this kind of modification in the usual physiological and psychological burn response can not only speed recovery and decrease suffering, it can save lives. When burns affect vital tissues or initiate shock, the relatively simple communication strategies that have been presented, combined with directives that produce images of being cool and comfortable can make a significant difference in survivability. This knowledge would be especially useful for fire fighters, for obvious reasons. And, since the effect requires the communication immediately after the injury, first responders have the greatest opportunity for making a difference in treatment outcome.

Situation:
A forty-eight-year-old male was driving a tractor when it broke an underground gas pipe, and a spark ignited a jet of gas. The driver sustained 24 percent total body surface second-degree burns. Rescuers are on the scene within fifteen minutes of receiving the call from the man's wife. After initial assessment, sterile dress-ings are applied to the surface burns; oxygen is administered; sufficient confidence, rapport, and expectations are developed within several minutes of arrival, using several strategies. The rescuer gives the following directive while applying the sterile dressing:

OK Mr. Brown. Do you know how to take care of this burn? [The patient admits that he does not.] Well, I do. But you can help me by thinking some happy thoughts, be-cause, believe it or not, I can treat you better when you do. Now you seem angry about the fact that you didn't know about the gas pipe location before you started work. It seems like an honest mistake to me. Besides, I think you've already been hurt enough with this accident, don't you?

Note that directives to eliminate guilt are especially useful for burn patients since very often the burn is a result of some negli-gent act. The rescuer continues.

Now, while we are preparing you for transport to the hospital, I want you to close your eyes for just a moment and imagine that, as I place the sterile gauze on your injuries, I am really packing the entire area in soft, clean snow. Remember what it was like to put your arm into a wall of very soft, very fresh, fallen snow? Notice how cool and comfortable each area is becoming as you see the snow being applied. Good.

The rescuer repeats this kind of image-producing dialogue several times. Remember that repetition helps the subconscious learn, but only up to a point. Generally, repeating the directive three to four times is sufficient. After that, there can be a tendency for the repetitive statement to cause a sense of urgency that activates analytic thinking at the expense of imagery thinking. Thus, after repeating the cool and comfortable imagery several times, the rescuer changes the focus as follows:

Good. Just allow that cool, comfortable feeling to continue on its own while we put you in the ambulance. Just concentrate on your right calf muscle, and see how relaxed it can become if you first tighten the muscle and then relax it. Go ahead and try that now. Good. Now just move that feeling of relaxation up through the rest of your body for the remainder of the ride to the hospital.

Note that the calf muscle is an uninjured part of the body. By focusing the patient's attention on relaxing an uninjured portion of the body, two things are accomplished. First, the directive for keeping the burn injury cool and comfortable until it heals is sealed in the subconscious as the rescuer matter-of-factly goes on to another subject. Second, the relaxation response that comes from tightening, then relaxing, an uninvolved muscle will in itself augment the psychological relaxation that will help calm and reassure the patient during transport.

Besides images of the snow, note that a cool mist of water, a cool, clean brook, a shady breeze, and so on can be used. Whenever possible, use the images that the patient tells you best bring about cool and comfortable feelings.

Remember to add to your cool-and-comfortable-directives words that imply cleanliness, freshness, and so on. This may augment the mind-body's natural tendency to heal wounds treated in this manner without risk of infection. Also, try to avoid using the word *normal* in your communication. In other words, do not say, "This is a common burn injury, and I expect you will have a normal reaction." A "normal" reaction is not what you are eliciting.

ENVIRONMENTAL EMERGENCIES

Besides thermal burns, chemical burns and sunburns can also be treated with the cool-and-comfortable directive. In the video, "Effective Communication with the Sick and Injured," available through Motivational Seminars, 205 San Marin Drive, Suite #2, Novato, California, 94945, Dr. Gerald Kaplan describes the use of this procedure with his son who suffered bad sun exposure after falling asleep at the beach. He directed him to imagine his face remaining cool and comfortable. The next day his face was not burned; however, his ears were. After considering what happened, Dr. Kaplan speculated that his son had not construed his ears to be a part of his face.

Other environmental emergencies due to heat exposure include heat cramps, heat exhaustion, and heat stroke. In each case the heat regulatory mechanisms are overwhelmed enough to cause a breakdown. While administering standard field treatment for each of these problems, simple directives can slow down or temporarily reverse the breakdown process.

The skin is especially influenced by psychological determinants. Hives, blushing, goose pimpling, and so on are all common emotional reactions. The skin, the largest single organ of the body, also serves to regulate the temperature of the body and to transmit information from the environment to the brain. Nerve endings that lie in the skin perceive and transmit information about heat, cold, pain, pleasure, and so on. As with any illness or injury, an overreactive vicious circle can begin when negative images from past experiences are triggered. Although physical cooling or hydration is extremely important, the capability of psychological cooling should not be neglected.

Situation:
A fifty-five-year-old female was hiking on a hot day in a state park in California. Park personnel were informed that she had fallen down on the trail and was complaining of dizziness and nausea. The rescuer responds and establishes a positive rapport. Expectations are built during initial assessment. The patient is alert, and she is given water to drink and placed in the shock position. Diagnosis is heat exhaustion. The rescuer tells her the following:

Mrs. Donnely, you can constrict or dilate your skin's blood vessels more or less when you need to. This means you can make them larger or smaller. This is a subconscious mechanism that you may not be aware of. It would be helpful, however, for you to imagine that your nervous system is directing just the right amount of dilation to help

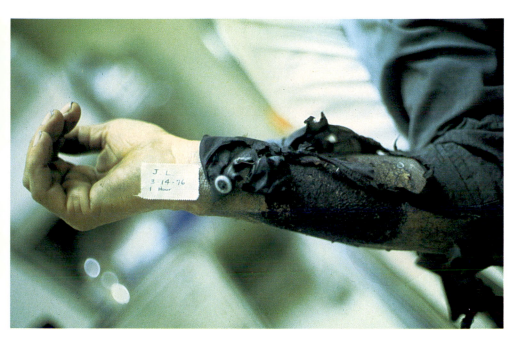

1: Patient's arm within one hour of being burned by an acetylene torch. Cool towels and suggestions for "cool and comfortable" were all that were given.

2: First dressing applied at 21 hours post burn. Dressing was applied over charcoal. No scrubbing was done.

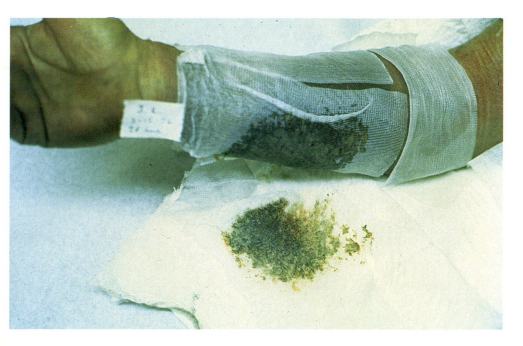

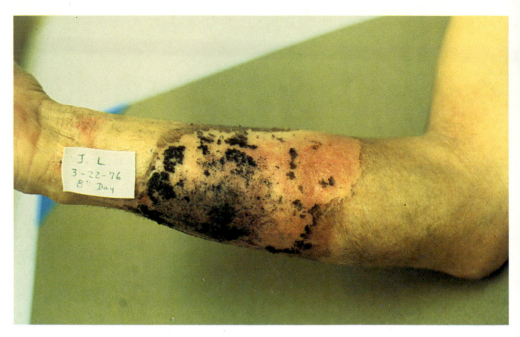

3: Arm at eight days. Healthy skin is beginning to appear.

4: Arm in 12 days. The arm has healed with no scar tissue.

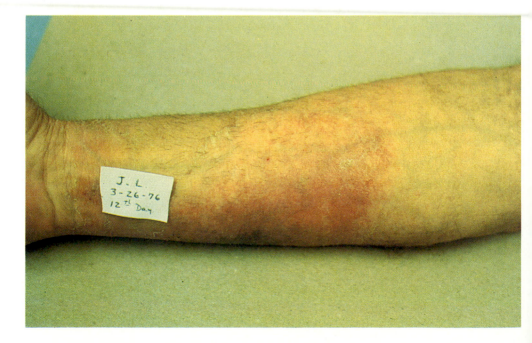

keep your body temperature at a safe level. Go ahead, now, and, in your own way, see or feel yourself responding positively to this need. Notice how your blood vessels are doing just exactly what they need to in order to keep you as cool and comfortable as is necessary.

Note that this directive does not use a metaphor like snow or cool water, although it would be fine to do so. Research has shown, however, that once the mind gets the main idea of the image, regulatory systems know what to do to implement the idea. Whether or not you use such a direct suggestion or use a more descriptive metaphor depends on which one you believe will work best for the particular patient.

Situation:
A man whose car ran out of gas attempted to walk along the Arizona desert freeway to find a gasoline station. After several hours of walking, he collapsed on the side of the road. A passerby stops, notes that the man's skin is very hot, dry, and flushed. He parks the car so as to place the man in the shade, then flags down another vehicle that goes for help. Neither car has water available. The passerby speaks to the man.

Listen to me. Help is on the way. For now, it is very important that you become as cool as possible. You can do this now by doing exactly what I say. Will you do what I say? [Patient indicates that he will.] Good. Now, when I count to three, I want you to see yourself, in your mind's eye, plunging into a very cold lake. You are wearing a life preserver, and there is nothing for you to do but to enjoy the cold, comfortable, refreshing sensation of the water. One, two, three. Now, feel and see yourself plunging into that cold lake. Notice how your body temperature is already beginning to lower. Good. Now, maintain that temperature and that feeling while we wait for the ambulance. Good. You're doing fine.

COLD EXPOSURE

Hypothermia is also a danger when temperature mechanisms react to extreme environmental conditions—in this case, cold. The rate and amount of heat loss by the body can be modified through a variety of metabolic systems that are controlled by the nervous system and that can be triggered by directives.

Ski patrol rescuers have reported finding patients who survived a night on cold mountain trails without proper protection. In some cases, patients stated that they were able to stay warm by *imagining* that they were in a warm place. Though the author has no specific case studies to refer to of rescuers giving warming suggestions to frightened patients of hypothermia, it is recommended that directives be given to such patients during standard treatment protocols.

EXERCISE

You arrive at the emergency scene and find a ten-year-old child who has been scalded by hot water. Write what you would say to the child, using a strategy for gaining rapport, a strategy for building positive expectation, and appropriate guidelines for an effective directive.

14 | Respiratory Distress

*This chapter answers the question of how to talk to
someone who is having trouble breathing.*

*B*reath is life. It is no wonder that patients suffering from acute respiratory disorders experience fear and panic. Fear and panic themselves affect breathing patterns. For example, hyperventilation associated with emotional states is relatively common. The person with labored breathing thus creates a vicious cycle, spiraling ever downward. With proper communication strategies, this cycle can be broken. Furthermore, the initial bronchospasm characteristics of many respiratory problems can effectively be controlled with suitably presented directives.

ASTHMA

When a person is having an asthma attack, a life-threatening emergency exists in that person's mind. A study done at the Walter Reed Allergy Department concluded that about 70 percent of asthmatic patients are absolutely frightened for breath during an attack. The patient's entire attention is concentrated on the next breath. For this reason, it is often difficult for the rescuer to get the patient's attention sufficiently to gain rapport and give appropriate directives unless the joining-in strategy is used in the following manner.

> *Situation:*
> *A thirty-six-year-old housewife is in the throes of an asthma attack when the rescuer arrives at the woman's home. She is sitting on a kitchen chair, desperately gripping the chair arms while she struggles for each breath. The rescuer approaches the patient so that her face is near the face of the patient. The rescuer then begins to mimic the labored breathing rate of the patient while talking.*

June, listen . . . to . . . me. It's really . . . hard to get . . . a breath, . . . isn't it? And . . . I know . . . how frightening that can be. But notice . . . just notice . . . that it is beginning to get . . . a bit easier now.

> *At this point, the rescuer's breathing begins to sound less labored. In most cases the patient's own breathing rate will begin to keep pace with the rescuer's. As the breathing rates become slower, the rescuer acknowledges the improvement with comments such as "Good," "That's fine," and so on.*

June, I have some pure, fresh oxygen for you that will help even more. As you inhale the oxygen, notice how much more relaxed your bronchioles become when you exhale."

[When giving the oxygen, the rescuer avoids placing the mask directly on the patient's face, as this might increase the anxiety.]

The standard treatment to be given by prehospital care personnel includes the administration of oxygen. If oxygen is available, the joining-in strategy can be used while it is being set up. In many instances, the patient will regain normal breathing even before the oxygen is administered. In any event, to enhance the benefit of the oxygen and to prevent further anxiety resulting from administering the oxygen, proper communication is also important.

Once the rescuer gets the patient's attention and has gained a positive rapport with the joining-in strategy, a specific directive to relax the muscles around the bronchi upon exhalation can be given to the asthma patient if the dyspnea continues.

Research at the Walter Reed Hospital in Washington, D.C., has shown that such specific directives have actual physiological effects on the bronchial tubes. In the research, participants inhaled a chemical that brings on an asthma attack. Measurements of forced exhalation were taken with and without directives. Directives given to participants during hypnotic states of consciousness resulted in significant increases in exhalation volume, revealing that the directives had a direct physiological influence on the bronchioles that were in spasm.

June, your breathing . . . is . . . becoming a little . . . easier now because you are beginning to *let* the muscles around your bronchi relax as you exhale. Just *continue* . . . to *allow* . . . those muscles to relax. That's good. You know, most people think that when you wheeze you can't get air into the lungs, but you and I know differently. We know it's just the opposite. When you are having an attack, you can't get the air out of the lungs to let fresh air in *until* you allow the bronchi muscles to relax as you are doing now. Just like your hand would open if you held a hot potato instead of closing, when you breathe in the oxygen, your bronchioles open up when they are full of oxygen.

In addition, to relieve the asthma attack at the emergency scene, the rescuer has an opportunity to explain to the asthma sufferer that they have the ability to "turn off" their wheezing anytime they need to. It can be explained that anyone suffering from asthma has simply developed a sensitivity to some irritant, possibly including biochemicals produced during emotional stress. The result is a learned response that triggers a complex of processes that cause mucus production and bronchospasm. Just as the nervous system has learned to respond to these sensitivities, it can also learn to stop the response, just as it did during the emergency call. In many cases, this comparatively simple and brief postemergency dialogue will prevent severe asthma attacks from ever occurring again. This is especially true when the patient is a child.

HYPERVENTILATION

Hyperventilating patients are also terrified of dying and have the feeling that it is impossible to get enough air into the lungs, in spite of the fact that they actually have breathed in too much oxygen. The immediate objective of the rescuer is to calm the patient and to raise the level of arterial carbon dioxide. Although this can be done effectively by having the patient rebreathe exhaled air from a paper bag, effective communication at the scene can also make a significant contribution to patient response and treatment outcome.

> *Situation:*
> *A twenty-four-year-old woman began hyperventilating after receiving news that her father had passed away. On arrival at the scene, the rescuer diagnoses that the patient is having a panic attack and that the symptoms are a result of simple overbreathing.*

> Joan, slow your breathing down *now*. Exhale on my count only! One, two, three. That's better. Joan, I know how frightened you are, and how upset you must be, but you will feel better soon. Right now you have inhaled too much oxygen, even though it seems like you aren't getting enough. By breathing into and out of this bag, you can balance out just the right amount of oxygen in your system and will feel better immediately. Go ahead and breathe into the bag, and notice how much more relaxed you are beginning to feel.

Notice that, for this emergency patient, an authoritarian, commanding approach is appropriate at the outset, followed by a more compassionate, understanding statement. This is usually the best way to gain rapport and give directives to a person suffering a panic attack.

CHOKING (PARTIAL AIRWAY OBSTRUCTION)

Many emergency situations arise when an airway is partially obstructed by some substance, such as a piece of meat. Since standard medical treatment is to avoid back blows or Heimlich maneuvers as long as the patient is able to exchange some air, communication is important for preventing respiratory distress from accelerating because of fear.

Situation:
A forty-nine-year-old male has choked on a piece of meat in a restaurant. When the rescuer arrives on the scene, the patient is gasping desperately for breath and people are gathered around him. While supporting the airway in its most efficient position, the rescuer projects confidence, gains rapport, and builds expectations before giving specific directives. The rescuer speaks slowly and calmly:

OK, Sir. I'm a paramedic, and you're going to be all right. It looks like you've got a piece of food started down the wrong pipe. I'm going to give you some pure oxygen [if available] that will help you feel better until we can get it out. In the meantime I want you to do as I say. Will you do that? [Rescuer makes a direct contract.] Good. Now I want you to just continue as you are doing because right now you are getting enough oxygen. When we get you to the hospital the docs can remove the food easily, and you'll be good as new. I'm not going to try myself because I don't want to get it lodged to where it stops the exchange of air you are *now* able to achieve.

The patient is now prepared for the following directive:

Now, I want you to imagine that you are sipping your oxygen through a straw, getting just enough to enjoy the quality of the air and to sustain your vital systems. Remain in as comfortable a position as you choose, and sip, rather than try to gulp, that air slowly, savoring every drop. Good. Now, notice how efficiently your body is able to utilize such small quantities of oxygen. And, notice how much easier it is for you to breathe even now through the small opening you are sipping your air through. Good.

EXERCISE

Using creative imagery of your own design, describe what you could say to a person with asthma that would help her visualize her breathing becoming more comfortable.

Miracle is the pet child of faith.
—Goethe

15 | Anaphylaxis

This chapter describes how words and thoughts can affect allergic reactivity in patients.

Although respiratory distress is a major concern when treating the patient with an anaphylactic reaction, a variety of nervous system responses to this problem can also be influenced via rescuer-patient communication.

Anaphylaxis is a fairly common emergency that can be life threatening. It occurs when someone has been sensitized to some substance at some point in time and then reacts violently to a subsequent contact. Offending agents include drugs (especially penicillin), certain foods and chemicals, and the sting of an insect.

In essence, the cause of an anaphylactic reaction is a hypersensitive immune system response to some foreign substance. The system somehow learned to be overprotective in defending the body against any future invasions from a one-time intruder. Exactly why the mind-body complex chooses to develop antibodies for a specific substance more aggressively than for another is not known. Emotional factors, however, at the time of the initial exposure, may be involved.

REDIRECTING THE IMMUNE SYSTEM

Directives given by a confident rescuer to a frightened emergency patient (who can be considered to be in a hypnotic state of consciousness) influence messages to and from the autonomic nervous system. The immune system is vitally connected to these messages. Research from Stanford, Mt. Sinai, and other medical research facilities has shown experimentally that the development of antibodies is closely associated with psychological processes, especially those interpreted as being stressful. Thus, the communication objective of the rescuer responding to an anaphylactic reaction emergency is to redirect the overreaction of the immune system to the specific antigen.

In addition to giving directives that can reverse bronchospasm, the other following signs of anaphylaxis should be reversed or stopped:

1. Inflammation and itching of the skin (hives)

2. Inflammation and edema in the larynx

3. Dilation of blood vessels and capillaries (reducing the amount of fluid in the vessels)

4. Continual release of the chemical, histamine, that causes the above condition

Before giving a sample narrative of directives that might achieve these objectives, it may be worthwhile to use this particular medical emergency to reiterate how your words can have such a profound effect on these very complex biochemical and physiological responses.

"MEMORY" IN THE IMMUNE SYSTEM

As has been stated, the anaphylactic reaction is a result of a previous learned association with some substance or antigen. In most cases, the antigen itself is relatively harmless. Nonetheless, the body will attack the substance with all its might when the substance is introduced into the bloodstream, even though the attack itself could cause death to the body.

If the mind-body complex learns to develop antibodies to attack certain antigens, we can infer that it has a "memory." Sometimes a subsequent exposure to an antigen occurs years after the initial exposure. Since memory implies images, even if at the cellular level, then we can begin to understand why words that form images might influence memory responses. Certainly this is the case at the psychological level, where new programs can be imagined that replace older ones. But only recently is research revealing that such memories, programs, or images exist at cellular or even microscopic levels throughout the mind-body system.

A fascinating example of this research was published in the June 1988 issue of the prestigious British journal, *Nature*. A French immunologist, Jacques Benveniste, took a common antibody (IgE) and exposed it to certain white cells in the blood called *basophils*. When this is done, the IgE typically attaches itself to certain receptor sites on the cells and waits to attack an antigen. The experiment began when Dr. Benveniste mixed the blood serum containing the white cells and IgE with a solution prepared from goat's blood that contained an anti-IgE (antigen). Dr. Benveniste knew that this would cause the antibody (IgE) to set off an allergic response resulting in the release of histamine.

So far, this was nothing new. Then Benveniste diluted the anti-IgE goat blood mixture tenfold and added it again to the human blood. The same reaction occurred. He kept on diluting, time after time, until the anti-IgE solution was diluted so drastically that it contained 1 part antibody to 10^{120} parts water. Mathematically, at this point, it was impossible for the water to contain a single molecule of antibody. The solution, however, which was basically now just distilled water, continued to set off the histamine reaction!

The experiment was duplicated seventy times by Benveniste and by researchers in Israel, Canada, and Italy. All came up with the same result. Was some kind of memory in the human white cells reacting to some infinitely small imprint? No one can say, and the experiment has stirred much controversy. But let us look at a more subjective example of how memory perception can trigger such reactions.

In his book, *Quantum Healing*, Dr. Deepak Chopra relates a story about his father and mother. His father, a cardiologist in India, was once stationed as an army doctor in a place called Jammu. His mother suffered there with severe asthma and anaphylactic reactions to the pollen of a native flower that blossomed every spring. (Could it be that her first visit there was accompanied by negative emotions since the place was so far from their home?) To avoid this, every spring his father drove his mother to Kashmir, where the air was free of this particular pollen and where she was delighted by the beauty of the mountain valley.

One spring the heavy rains had made the road impassable for the return trip to Jammu, so they chartered an airplane and returned home early. When the plane landed, the mother's skin began to welt and blister, and she had difficulty breathing. When the steward ran up to her, the father said, "There's nothing you can do. It's the pollen in Jammu."

The steward looked puzzled and explained that they had not yet landed in Jammu, but at Udhampur, their first stop. Within moments, Chopra's mother stopped struggling for breath, and her sores vanished on the spot.

Similar to this story, many multiple-personality cases have been studied where the patient's personality shifts also change physiological characteristics. One personality can be color blind, another normal. One personality can have diabetes; the other does not. One personality can have hypertension; as soon as another personality appears, the hypertension disappears! No one can yet explain these things, but as some sense of a quantum memory that can be modified when image responsive chemicals receive new pictures of reality. Language may be a control switch that initiates this phenomenon.

Situation:
A twenty-two-year-old female, allergic to bee stings, was stung in the neck while gardening. She immediately called the fire department. Within minutes the fire department arrives on the scene and finds the patient with swelling about the lips and tongue, red and itching skin, and stomach cramps. The patient is anxious and complains that the reaction is going to get much worse.

After accomplishing the credibility, rapport, and expectation objectives indicated by the first three letters of the CREDIBLE

mnemonic (while the stinger is removed and oxygen is adminis-
tered), the following directive is given by the rescuer while wait-
ing for the paramedics.

Sally, I want you to listen to me carefully now. Have you
ever gotten goose pimples on your skin after thinking
about something exciting or scary? Did they stay and get
worse, or did they go away when you stopped thinking
about them? [Patient responds that they went away.] Well,
your reaction to the bee sting is similar to the goose bump
reaction. The stinger is out and the substance has dissipated into your bloodstream. Your body has forgotten how
to turn off the reaction. But you can do that now. I just
want you to imagine that those antibodies that keep pro-
ducing the chemicals making your skin red and swollen
have been called off. They have been thanked for trying
their best to attack the bee venom but were told that they
were much more aggressive than they needed to be. And,
now that the venom has been dissipated in your bloodstream, they can stop and allow your body to return to a
cool and comfortable state.

Just begin to feel your blood vessels constricting again
and see in your mind's eye all the chemical processes that
started a few minutes ago beginning to reverse. Notice that
your throat and face are beginning to feel cooler and more
comfortable already.

I have personally used this communication with several similar
cases and have witnessed remarkable cessation of the severe reactions that could have led into shock. In fact, I used this approach on
myself once and believe that it saved my life.

My wife and I were traveling in Peru. Circumstances forced us
to be in the streets of Lima after curfew, but the political clout of a
stranger brought us safely to our hotel. When we arrived there, the
bar was still open, and our new friend invited us to sample the native
drink, Pisco Sours. Courtesy dictated that we did not refuse. Though
not an accomplished drinker, I managed to finish the four drinks I
was given. At 3:00 A.M. my wife and I climbed into our bed. Within
ten minutes my throat began to itch and my skin began to burn. Then
everything began to swell. With the swelling came pain and fear. We
were in the middle of Lima during curfew. Americans were not
favored by the government. The hotel did not house physicians.
Whatever was happening to me, it was up to me to survive.

When my larynx began to close, I knew I was having a severe anaphylactic reaction—probably to whatever was in the Pisco Sours. With that realization, I began to concentrate on survival. As a result of my research into the subject of this book, I had confidence in my imagery capabilities. In fact, I had just recently undergone an appendectomy without local or general anesthesia. (An interesting footnote to that experience is that I felt the incision cutting my abdominal wall vertically because that was how I imagined they were going to do it. Not until after the operation did I see that the incision was made horizontally.) Nonetheless, the intense pain and narrowing larynx challenged my confidence tremendously.

Once my wife accepted that I was in control, she patiently continued to place cool towels on my swollen extremities. I was soon in a hypnotic state of consciousness, and I began to give myself directives similar to the following:

> OK, Don, you are having an allergic reaction to something you ate or drank tonight. You know that this response is an over-reaction and can be reversed. Some distorted memory of a past antigen is creating this havoc, and the control center in your mind can issue orders to put your body back in equilibrium. You are already beginning to notice your body chemistry responding positively.

I continued this kind of rhetoric for almost an hour before noticeable alleviation of swelling and itching took place. By 5:00 A.M., I was back to normal condition, save being exhausted.

The next day I asked the bartender what ingredients were in Pisco Sours. The translation in English was grain alcohol and raw egg whites. The raw egg whites rang a bell. For years I had been mildly allergic to raw egg whites. If I accidently undercooked my eggs or ate meringue, I would sniffle, my eyes would water, and my throat would scratch a little. The alcohol mixture must have intensified my response to the extreme. Had I not used my imagery capabilities to redirect the cellular memories of my immune system, I very well could have died in that Peruvian hotel.

POISON OAK

Although poison oak or ivy reactions do not often constitute an emergency crisis, they do occasionally. Even less serious cases can cause a great deal of suffering. In his 1968 book, *Clinical Hypnotherapy*, Dr. David Cheek states in the concluding remarks of his chapter

"Emergency Uses and Spontaneous Trance," "Emergency uses of hypnosis are numerous and the valuable possibilities obvious with such urgent situations as highway accidents, burns, cardiac arrest, surgical shock, status asthmaticus, and any crisis where a patient seems to have lost motivation toward recovery. We have not explored all the ways in which a body can cope with cancer, with acute dermatitis like poison oak."

I had remembered the mention of poison oak once when a fire fighter came to me immediately after extinguishing a wildland fire in which he inhaled much smoke from burning poison oak. He appeared desperate and told me that he had had to be hospitalized the last time he contacted poison oak on a hike. He felt sure that handling the hose that was pulled through the bushes and breathing in the smoke would result in a catastrophic and disabling reaction.

With a sound of matter-of-factness in my voice, I assured him that the response to poison oak was an autonomic nervous system action that could easily be modified with a new inner belief system. He was frightened enough to be hypersuggestible to what I was saying, and it was therefore unnecessary to hypnotize him formally. I asked him to get comfortable in a chair and to tell his body that *this* time he would only experience a mild rash. I told him that he would be able to see the rash, but that it would be so comfortable he would not feel it. The next morning he came to me overjoyed. A mild red rash appeared on his arms, belly, and neck. He claimed that there was no itching.

Since this case, many people, including my wife, have been able to radically modify their reactive responses to poison oak with directives that create friendly images relating to the plant, rather than hostile or defensive ones.

In an emergency situation, the same approach can be used for acute poison oak or ivy reaction as was illustrated for anaphylaxis.

EXERCISE

You have a patient allergic to bee sting who has been stung on the foot by a yellow jacket. Ten minutes have elapsed, and the swelling is increasing steadily. You are with the patient during transport to the hospital. What would you say to keep the person from going into shock?

16 | Childbirth and Pediatric Emergencies

Children are not only easily influenced by your manner and words during a traumatic experience; their response to future traumas is also in your hands. This chapter illustrates proper communication strategies with children and with women during emergency childbirth.

CHILDBIRTH EMERGENCIES

In the past twenty years, many training programs preparing pregnant women for an efficient, painfree birth experience have come forth. Most of these programs teach the husband to communicate effectively with his wife during labor, reminding her to concentrate on remaining calm, positive, and happy. The training exercises, each in their own way, teach women to induce a trance in herself by focusing upon breathing patterns, movement of the arms, and muscle relaxation. The process is pictured as a work and rest cycle, and the mother is encouraged to see the entire experience as a wonderful, not a painful, event.

If there are no complications to disrupt the concentration, and if the breathing and relaxation techniques have been mastered, the outcome is as nature intended. Toxic analgesics and drugs are not needed. This, and the reduced stress on both mother and child, make it possible for the mother to assist in the process of childbirth with reasonable comfort. It also allows for the mother (and father) to relate immediately to the newborn baby.

Unfortunately, many women do not take advantage of such training programs. Even when they do, deeply ingrained perceptions regarding pain or inappropriate language between nurses and physicians at the hospital can change the wonderful birth experience to a stressful, painful event. With what you now know about the power of words, imagine how you would feel as a pregnant mother entering the hospital and hearing the paramedic tell the nurse, "Her *labor pains* are starting to occur more often and last longer."

When a mother's plans to be safe at the hospital during labor somehow become upset and the birth begins elsewhere, fear can negatively affect the outcome. Pain, hemorrhage, toxemia, and even infection have been associated with the undue stress and fear during labor. With the CREDIBLE mnemonic's communication approach, however, we have a way to offer hope, stop hemorrhage, reduce pain, reverse the effects of toxemia, and improve resistance to infection.

As someone responding to a childbirth situation, your first priority is to project confidence, establish positive rapport, and build hopeful expectations with the mother. Any of the strategies presented in the earlier chapters can be used to accomplish these three objectives. Subsequent directives are also intended to dispel worries and fears. Even when there are serious complications, assurances that positive outcomes are likely can make all the difference.

Situation:

A twenty-four-year-old woman is in her first stage of labor. The amniotic sac ruptured moments after the rescuer arrived on the scene. Ambulance service is too far away, so the family station wagon is used to transport the mother to the hospital, which is thirty minutes away. This will be the woman's second pregnancy; her first child aborted at six months. The rescuer has attained good rapport with the mother, and sterile supplies for delivery are ready in case birth happens before reaching the hospital. The rescuer gives her positive reassurances:

There is only one thing that is important now, that your delivery be a wonderful experience for you. Your delivery is going to be *reasonably comfortable,* and you are going to have your baby with a great big smile on your face. In fact, even if you wanted to, you wouldn't be able to keep from smiling the moment your baby is born.

Whether your baby is born here in the car or at the hospital does not matter. In either case your delivery is going to be a wonderful experience, and that smile is going to show it.

At any point along the way you might become temporarily distracted from your *comfortable effort.* That's quite all right, because you will immediately return to focus on that comfortable effort that we call labor. You can do this because the only thing that is really on your mind is the fact that, in a little while, you will be seeing the wonderful baby you've been waiting for. There is nothing to bother. Nothing that can interfere with your having your baby as quickly and easily as possible.

In many cases, the woman involved in an emergency childbirth will have a relatively optimistic attitude on her own. The above directives serve to maintain this optimism throughout the many worries and annoyances that might occur during the labor. In some cases, however, the woman will be entering the labor without this optimism. Instead, worry, fear, and even guilt are dominant emotions. Women who are unhappy with their pregnancy and/or are afraid of the pain and possible complication they *believe* to be probable can create some of the problems listed earlier. Although the above directive may suffice to alleviate such concerns, a more direct approach may be more effective *if* you know in advance just what those concerns are.

To find out what these fears are, you could simply ask the woman, "Do you have any worries, concerns, or fears about your delivery?" Unfortunately, this question might cause the patient without such problems to think of some. According to David Cheek, to ask directly is to suggest the expectation that pregnant women should be afraid. Dr. Cheek, a diplomate of the American Board of Obstetrics and Gynecology, has pioneered much of the research that associates psychological states during pregnancy and labor with a variety of physical and mental responses.

According to Dr. Cheek, the best way to find out if a pregnant woman has a sufficiently healthy attitude about giving birth is with ideomotor responses regarding the sex of the unborn child. If the woman commits herself to a decision, his research shows that it is likely that the attitude is positive. If the response indicates, I don't know, or I don't want to answer, it is probably that some fear is at work.

Setting up the ideomotor response is any easy thing to do with the woman in labor. Here is an example:

> Mary, I want you to go ahead and concentrate on those deep, relaxing breaths. In the meantime, I want to ask you a few questions using a technique that won't interrupt your concentration. The only answers you need to give me are yes, no, or I don't know, which can also mean, I don't want to answer. Just slightly raise your index finger [indicate which hand] for yes, your second finger for no, and your thumb for I don't know, or I don't want to answer. If you understand, let me know by raising the correct finger. Good.

At this point the rescuer can ask some simple history questions or other questions that can easily lead into the opportunity to ask about the baby's sex.

- OK, is this your first pregnancy?

- Does the moist towel on your forehead still feel cool?

- Is someone going to meet you at the hospital?

- I'm curious as to what sex you think your baby is going to be. Is it going to be a boy? A girl?

If the thumb raises, according to Cheek, a fear exists as indicated by the unwillingness to make a commitment to making a decision. The source of the fear is usually some ridiculous identification originating in reading material, television, or conversations with well-meaning friends and relatives that have produced images about giving birth being an ordeal. There might also be financial concerns, relationship problems, and so on. In any event, if the thumb responds, you can then continue with more direct interrogations about a potential fear by asking, "Are there any worries, fears, or concerns that are troubling you now?" If the response is "no," just accept the answer and continue with the directives presented earlier. If the response is either "yes," or "I don't know," then it is usually quite easy to expose the problem and resolve the fear with a few reassuring sentences that help dilute the concern. Once accomplished, return to the original directive and repeat it. According to Cheek, if you have indeed resolved the concern sufficiently, you could ask the question again regarding the probable sex of the child and the woman would this time let you know if she thinks the baby is a boy or a girl.

PEDIATRIC EMERGENCIES

The first responder attending a child suffering from a medical emergency has a special opportunity. Not only can his actions and words help save the child from a permanent, disabling injury, but they can significantly influence the child's response to future injuries or illnesses, as well as to future interventions by medical personnel. Furthermore, of all age groups, children are the most impressionable and generally have the greatest capacity for visual imagery. Once a positive rapport with a child is attained, little to no preparation is necessary to go right into what might be considered dramatic directives.

Because of this extreme suggestibility to words and the images they create, it is especially important to monitor or prevent well-intended but potentially damaging remarks from concerned relatives. If such remarks are heard by the child, simply rephrasing them so the child can interpret them positively can reverse the negative effects quickly. This also serves to educate the parent to leave the communication to you. When establishing rapport with a child, it is important to remember that a stranger, especially a uniformed one, alone may be frightening. This is the opposite of the effect a uniformed rescuer has on most injured adults. The older a child is, of course, the more likely he will also respond positively to the rescuer. In any event, establishing a positive rapport is usually easy when the joining-in strategy is used at the outset.

The joining-in strategy works so well to get children and adolescents into your confidence because most adults tend to alienate them with their language. Statements like the following usually do not create rapport:

- Come on, Johnny, it's not that bad.
- Don't be a crybaby.
- Everything is fine. Don't worry.
- You be brave now, and the fireman will give you a ride in his fire truck.

Johnny probably does think his hurt arm is bad. Crying feels natural to him. He does not want to be called names. He knows everything is not fine. And, he could care less about bravery and a ride in the fire truck at this point. What he would prefer to hear from an adult is an acknowledgment of what he is really feeling and thinking, even if it is not constructive. The rescuer who approaches the scene, introduces himself, and says, "Boy, I'll bet that really hurts, and I bet it's scary being out here with all these people standing around, huh?" will gain quicker rapport.

Now the child has found someone in whom he can trust. He will listen to directives that gradually reframe his interpretation of the situation. The following is another example.

Well, it looks like you cut yourself. I'll bet that really hurts. And look at all that blood. Look at that good, red, strong, healthy blood. You know, I'll bet that has bled just enough now to clean out the wound. You can go ahead and stop the bleeding now while I get you a bandage. OK. Good job.

In this example, the joining-in strategy was quickly followed by a reframing of the situation. The boy agreed with the statements and the tonation relating to "all that blood." He then agreed that the blood was "good" and "strong." And, he agreed that it had probably bled enough to do what it was supposed to do. Finally, he agreed that he could go ahead and stop the bleeding. After all, everything else the rescuer said was true.

The following case study illustrates just how many contributions to the child's future proper communication can make.

Situation:
A three-year-old female was left unattended for a few minutes. She walked to a kennel that contained six huskies bred for sled racing. One of the dogs knocked her down and the others jumped on her, biting and pawing at her (apparently in play). Her father heard her screams and rescued her from the dogs after several minutes. By then she had suffered a lacerated cornea, a ripped ear,

several puncture wounds on her legs, arms, and face, and a large avulsion on the back of her hand. The fire department was called and arrives within minutes. The little girl is screaming hysterically at that time. Upon approach, the rescuer lifts the child's hand and looks directly and only at the avulsion—this helps narrow the focus of the little girl to just one thing at the outset:

Oh, boy, I'll bet that hand really hurts. And look at how your skin is folded back like that. I'll bet you didn't know what your skin looked like underneath before. Well, do you know that that will feel more comfortable if you fold the skin back to where it was? [At this point the child is still crying, but she has paid enough attention to become interested in what the fire fighter is talking about.]

Why don't you go ahead and fold that skin back; then you can help me take care of your other sores. OK. Here, just use this sterile cloth and put the skin right back where it was. [He places the 4-by-4-inch bandage in her other hand.]

Good, now just lift right here and lay the skin flap right back down again. [The child stops crying and follows the instructions.]

From this point on, the child participates in treating all of the wounds that she can reach. Each one is talked about as though it is a special, important item. To keep the emphasis on the child remaining relatively painfree, a game is set up whereby the paramedic claims he can find the wound that "feels the best." When a more hurtful wound is discussed, it is quickly treated and the search for the "best" wound continues. By this time, less than five minutes from the start, the child is smiling and conversing freely.

Once the wounds are superficially treated, the rescuer begins discussing the dogs.

You know, I'll bet those dogs really feel sad about what they did. They are used to playing rough like that with each other. They just didn't know how to play with a little girl. I'll bet when you get your own dogs you can teach them how to play with you, can't you? [Response is positive.] Good. And, I'll bet you could even teach them how to play with little boys and girls if you are older when you get a dog. Huh? That's right.

With this simple communication, the likely chance of the child having a phobia about dogs in later years is probably reduced to zero.

When the ambulance arrives, the child is formally introduced to the paramedics. The paramedics are told exactly what happened to the girl. Then, much praise is given regarding her handling of the situation and her self-treatment of the wounds. The little girl is told by the original rescuer that she will truly like the paramedics because they know a lot about how to get injuries like hers to heal quickly. She is also told that the doctors and nurses at the hospital will do things that will help the wounds heal more quickly. To both of these directives is added the phrase, "of course, you'll have to help them like you helped me."

At the end of the twenty minutes of treatment and communication with this patient, positive programs are recorded in her mind that will affect her attitude about emergency personnel, doctors, injuries, healing, dogs, and helping others for perhaps the rest of her life. Not bad for a day's work. And is not that what being a rescuer is all about?

In another case, a different approach to pain control is used after rapport is gained. In this situation the imagery capabilities of the child are more directly brought into play.

Situation:
A twelve-year-old boy was badly beaten on virtually all parts of his body by his father. When the father left the house, neighbors brought the child to the fire station. The child appeared to be suffering significant pain in numerous locations. After the confidence, rapport, and expectation aspects of the CREDIBLE mnemonic are handled, and the appropriate medical treatment and dispatch are complete (including a report of child abuse), the following directives for pain control are given.

Louis, I want you to close your eyes for a little while because I'm going to show you how to do something that will make you feel more comfortable. Now, as you close your eyes, you can let your whole body just go limp, just the way a wet towel does when you drop it on the floor.

This particular directive serves to assure that the child is in that state of consciousness that will indeed make him highly receptive to the pain control directives that will follow. This is done because of the time that elapsed between the actual beating and the visit to the fire station. Although the child is still frightened, the possibility that spontaneous hypersuggestibility may have relinquished itself to left brain thinking is there. Since children can quickly be brought back into this receptive state of consciousness with simple requests to imagine relaxing feelings, such a directive can always be used before more specific ones are given.

Good. Now I want you to imagine a long row of light switches. Above each switch is a colored bulb, all turned on, and each one a different color. There's a blue one and a yellow one and a green one. What other colors do you see? [The child answers "Yellow and red."] Good.

Now, these switches all have round knobs on them that allow you to turn down the light and make it dimmer. Or, you can turn it down all the way until the light is off.

This light system is very much like your own nervous system. Your nervous system sends messages to and from your brain to all the parts of your body. And it can turn down or turn off different feelings in the body.

Now, let me show you how this works. [At this point the rescuer assigns one of the light switches to an *uninjured* part of the body. In this case it is the child's left hand.] Imagine that your hand is connected to the blue light switch. Now start turning down the dimmer until the light is almost off. Notice that your hand is beginning to feel nice and comfortable. You can feel the pressure of my fingers when I touch it, but there is no discomfort when I pinch it. Go ahead and pinch it yourself now. Good.

Now, turn the blue light back on so you have normal feeling in that hand, and let's assign some light switches to places on your body where you would like to feel more comfortable.

After the switches are assigned, the child can turn down or turn off his pain anywhere he chooses very quickly.

Your own imagination is the only limit to the images that can be used to help children through medical emergencies. You will probably feel more comfortable using imagery with children than with adults as you begin to use the language of healing, so experiment with different images and directives. As long as you follow the rules outlined in earlier chapters, you cannot go wrong. And, you will have given much more to the child than a bandage and a ride to the hospital.

TRUE OR FALSE?

1. Women about to give birth seldom have any fears or anxieties that can make the event difficult.

2. Children involved in a medical emergency are not as receptive to suggestions as are adults.

3. The joining-in strategy is very effective with children.

4. The effectiveness of emergency treatment of young children can affect their reactions to future trauma.

When written in Chinese, the word crises is
composed of two characters. One represents danger
and the other represents opportunity.
—John F. Kennedy

17 | Psychological Crisis

A psychological injury can be as devastating as a
physical one. This chapter discusses several examples
and offers effective communication strategies for each.

*T*he word *crisis* is used to describe an emotional state of stress that can result in a radical change in a person's status. Although many emergency patients experience psychological crisis as a component of their physical injury or illness, this chapter is devoted to those cases where the emotional status alone is the basis for risk. In other words, the crisis is precipitated by primarily psychological difficulties. Examples common to emergency rescue include people affected by sudden death of a loved one, suicidal individuals, raped or abused victims, and extremely disruptive people.

In this type of crisis, the patient's capacity for initiative and self-direction may be severely impaired. In such a case, the rescuer can assume that the patient is completely psychologically dependent on his directives. As with most individuals in altered states of consciousness, however, directives cannot be successfully given until rapport is gained. This is especially challenging to the rescuer since, in these emergencies, patients have a limited potential for overt response at the time of the crisis. It is therefore more difficult to know when rapport has actually been achieved. With continual communication, the traumatized person will eventually become sufficiently attentive to your language. Once this has occurred, the opportunities for helping the patient regain control with your words and manner are significant.

SUDDEN DEATH OF A LOVED ONE

Each person responds so uniquely to the death of a loved one and each situation is so different that it is difficult to list general communication strategies. The following guidelines and case studies, however, do describe some consistently effective tactics.

First of all, the rescuer should realize that some type of emotional or physical response is a normal part of the grief process. Respect the grieving person's need for sympathy and follow her wishes if they seem relatively harmless. Sometimes this can be a difficult call. For example, I would let the wife of a man who has just died from a heart attack go to his side if she demanded it. I probably would not let a mother go to the side of her badly mutilated son, however.

It is also important to be truthful and direct with friends and relatives of individuals who have suddenly died. They will be hyper-intuitive about the facts, and indirect statements or partial truths will often disrupt rapport and trust. If you are asked, "Is he dead?" and you know he is, you have no choice but to tell the truth. Exceptions to this rule might include a situation where the news could significantly aggravate a medical condition.

Similarly, the rescuer should not speculate about the unknown. If the facts are uncertain, this should be admitted. By doing this, the rescuer and the patient enter into a bond, with both parties realizing that the future is a mystery to all. (Of course, if there is no doubt that the injured person is going to survive, then such information should be communicated.) By acknowledging the natural lack of omniscience that we all share, that helpless feeling the person in stress experiences diminishes with the realization that we are all somewhat helpless during such times.

As with children, the joining-in strategy with a progressive reframing of images is very effective. In the following case, the rescuer joins in and encourages the patient's overwhelming grief, then directs her toward calmness with pleasant images. It is important to allow for or encourage actual crying because crying serves as a catharsis for pain and tension. With crying, blood pressure at first goes up, but then it tends to lower afterward. Increased oxygenation also occurs during crying.

Situation:
A thirty-four-year-old woman and her seven-year-old son crashed their car into the side of a cliff on a winding road trying to avoid a deer. The car burst into flames on impact. The woman escaped unharmed, but could not reach through the flames to get her son out of the car. Several people passing by stopped to help. One person restrained the woman from going near the burning car while the other tried his best to open the door. By the time the fire department arrives, the boy is severely burned and obviously dead. The mother is hysterical and is calling for her boy. Several times she screams, "My God, he's burned to death!" The rescuer approaches the woman calmly and professionally, then firmly takes her by the arm and walks her two steps away from the crowd:

Ma'am, it's time to cry. Your son has passed away, and there's nothing we can do for him now but to remember him and cry. Let the other firemen do their job. I'll stay with you and help you. The worst is over now and you must remember how important it is for you to take care of your other children.

Throughout this communication the rescuer provides sincere support for the woman. He joins her in her grief. Sharing of the sadness in this way adds to the effectiveness of the joining-in strategy. The shared grieving causes the pain and suffering of the moment to diminish enough for her to regain control. As she begins to respond to the rescuer's questions, she also becomes ready to listen to directives that will lead her into the ambulance and away from the scene.

In many instances, relatives at the scene of an emergency suffer from psychological crisis at the onset of a medical crisis with a loved one, when death is feared but has not yet occurred. While first responders work on the medical patient, this person's behavior can be damaging to himself and to the primary patient who has become suddenly ill or injured. Joining in with this person's feelings and then gradually taking control of the feelings is again very effective. Simply acknowledging the distraught person's feelings can have a noticeable calming effect. Thus, instead of saying, "It's OK, he's going to be fine; just calm down," say, "You're real scared, but we are going to take good care of him."

This simple statement tends to build instant rapport. Once this is accomplished, a directive should be given that is meaningful to the person and that should partially distract her from the emotional trauma. For example, you can say, "I need you to help me take care of your husband. I need you to calm down, go to that corner, and wait for the ambulance."

SUICIDE ATTEMPTS

In the following case, the grieving wife of a man who died from a cocaine overdose attempted suicide while the medics were still on the scene. Although the man was dead, CPR efforts were initiated and could not be stopped (legally) until the paramedic team reached the hospital and the man was pronounced dead by a physician.

Situation:
One fire fighter remains in the area and returns to the house to check on the wife and obtain information for his report. He walks into the house and finds the woman collapsed on the floor. An empty bottle of phenobarbital pills lays at her side. Her respirations are failing, and her pulse rate is falling. After calling for another ambulance and mutual aid from another fire department, the fire fighter begins giving strategic directives to the unconscious woman while administering oxygen:

Mrs. Davis, listen to me. The worst is over now. Whatever has happened to your husband, there is still much for you to do. If you had any guilt about anything, that guilt is now leaving you. If you have any anger, that anger is leaving as well. Now you are going to be reborn into life for yourself. With each breath that passes through your lungs, your body will cleanse out the chemicals you took to gain relief from your grief. As these chemicals clear out, you will feel your health returning. Soon you will begin to feel a lightness inside yourself as you move along your rebirth and return to life. Let every part of your body respond to this lightness, or is it a brightness? With each breath passing through your lungs, feel the chemicals being cleansed out of your body. Notice the new feeling of harmony with friends and family. Let that bright lightness carry you into your rebirth and return to life.

The fire fighter repeats this kind of rhetoric for almost forty-five minutes, the time it takes for the next group of rescuers to arrive. By that time, Mrs. Davis has regained consciousness, and her vital signs are improving. Later, after he has pumped out her stomach, the hospital physician tells the fire fighter that the woman's recovery is remarkable.

RAPE

Victims of rape require significant emotional support that can be rapidly given with proper communication strategies. Whether the patient is withdrawn or hysterical, she should be treated with extreme gentleness and respect. Statements that reflect anger, disgust, or blame should be carefully avoided. The rescuer should not criticize the patient with comments such as, "You really shouldn't have been walking in this area," and so on. All words that are spoken should emphasize the fact that the worst is over. In such cases, this phrase can be so effective in calming and reassuring the patient that it can be helpful to ask her to repeat it to herself over and over again. By evoking her participation, either in repeating words you ask her to speak or by assisting in any first aid that may be necessary, the patient regains a sense of control that she desperately needs to reclaim.

DISRUPTIVE BEHAVIOR

Occasionally a first responder will come across an extremely disruptive individual whose behavior could harm himself or others, including the rescuer. The causes for such behavior are many. Alcohol and drug use are the most common. Certain physical and mental conditions, from concussions to diabetic shock also may be responsible. For some people, this kind of behavior is a normal reaction to stress. In any case, the first responder's first and safest treatment is with words and manner.

When dealing with this type of patient, avoid expressing your own anger or fear. Do not be heard using terms like *crazy* or *drunk*. Maintain a body posture that is nonaggressive. Even though you may be concerned for your own safety, avoid any action or statement that will make you "part of the enemy" or a target for the patient's violence.

The rapport strategy of choice with this kind of emergency is *feedback*, followed by a variation of the joining-in strategy. Speaking calmly, slowly, and directly to the patient, the rescuer should pay careful attention to what is being said. If the patient is not speaking, a question can be asked to elicit some statement. Whatever the patient says, the rescuer should wait a few moments, then feed back the same information. Then, the statement should be repeated, this time sounding as though the idea, thought, or feeling were the rescuer's own. In many instances, the statements will be negatively oriented toward someone. Nonetheless, the rescuer should continue the feedback and joining-in charade until a positive rapport is established with the patient. Then, subsequent directives can diffuse the violence and belligerence.

> *Situation:*
> *A thirty-two-year-old male left a bar with a revolver and began shooting in the air and threatening to kill someone named Fred. The man was obviously under the influence of alcohol. After he had used up all the bullets in the gun, he threw it on the ground and took a pocket knife out of his pocket. He then challenged anyone to take it out of his hands, while occasionally continuing to talk about putting an end to Fred. The man's behavior was borderline hysterical, and fits of crying were intermittent.*
>
> *Several of his friends had attempted to approach him, with no success, when an off-duty police officer, knowledgeable in effective communication strategies, steps several yards in front of the disruptive patient.*

Rescuer: What's your name?
Patient: None of your damned business!
Rescuer: It's hot out tonight. Listen, you probably think that it's none of my business what your name is. Right?
Patient: That's right. Who are you?
Rescuer: You know, it's none of my business who you are, and I don't even know what I am doing out here, but I am really feeling angry at that damned Fred.

At this point the rescuer has gained a rapport with the patient. Disruptive patients do not tend to remember the words or thoughts that they speak from one moment to the next, yet the feeling behind the words remains. Feeding back information and joining in agreement are thus effective tactics for "becoming friends" with the person, especially when the cause of disruption is alcohol or drug related. After the rapport is gained and dialogue exists between the two, the officer asks the man to walk away from the crowd so they can talk more. In a short while the patient is crying in the police officer's arms about the girl he lost to Fred.

EXERCISE

An eighteen-year-old boy just wrecked his father's car. Although he appears to have a broken arm, he will not allow anyone to come near him. He angrily threatens those around him. You are a paramedic in uniform and arrive at the scene. Develop a dialogue that might allow you to gain his confidence and direct him to compliance. Explain why you use the words you use.

18 | Saving Yourself

This chapter teaches how automatic responses to danger can be learned and that certain beliefs can be adopted that will enhance your ability to save yourself during a personal trauma.

*T*hus far we have concentrated on the task of saving others. But how can we influence our own involuntary nervous system so as to enhance personal survival? Can the communication strategies and techniques that work with our patients have any effect when we are using them on ourselves? How can we prepare ourselves to have optimal survival reactions during an emergency crisis?

STATE-DEPENDENT LEARNING

It is the patient's own imagery that ultimately makes a difference in treatment outcome. The rescuer's language merely stimulates those images. The patient produces the desired results by carrying out the ideas presented to her. If the emergency patient's thoughts are not properly guided, inappropriate images often cause vital functions to degenerate. However, if a person is prepared for the discomfort and unfamiliar circumstances associated with a critical injury, then she is in a position to initiate her own positive images.

Unfortunately, preparing for the unknown and unexpected is not as easy as memorizing a list of rules. Even when ideal responses are studied, they are likely to be forgotten when they are truly needed. A paramedic who has successfully utilized these communication strategies with many patients would likely be unable to maintain equal confidence if she had to contend with her own medical emergency.

In order to gain confident and positive control over nervous system functions during an emergency, mental processes must be programmed to react instantly and automatically. Such automatic responses require what is referred to as *state-dependent learning*. The theory of state-dependent learning argues that subconscious behavior can only be modified when the learning takes place during certain receptive states of consciousness, such as exists with waking or spontaneous hypnosis. Thus a child ordered to never touch a heater again at the moment he is burning his finger is more apt to permanently and automatically alter his behavior than the child that learns the same lesson in a classroom.

Learning what is not state-dependent can be implemented during normal circumstances but may be overridden by contrary state-dependent lessons during emotional stress. For example, a person accustomed to losing her temper when confronted by a rude person might have taken a course that taught her to simply ignore the antagonist and walk away. In spite of the fact that the lesson is well understood and accepted, when an actual incident occurs, it is probable that the old anger reflex will nonetheless prevail, unless this special state of consciousness existed while the new learning was happening.

To achieve the calm and reassuring attitude in an emergency that will facilitate control of autonomic nervous system functions requires practicing with self-hypnosis in the relative safety of your home or workplace. By using self-hypnosis, you can duplicate the state of consciousness automatically experienced by emergency patients when they are able to accept new images.

SELF-HYPNOSIS

Ultimately, all hypnosis is self-hypnosis. Although it is usually easier to allow a trained person to help direct appropriate images, the same results can be obtained by practicing self-hypnosis. Practicing with hypnosis during nonemergencies will prepare you for using it to advantage during a crisis.

As with patient communication in the field, a deep trance is not necessary for preparing the mind to cope with future crisis. In fact, a deep trance state often causes the tired individual to take advantage of the relaxation and fall asleep instead of maintaining the hypnotic state of consciousness.

Since by now you have acquired a thorough understanding of imagery phenomenon and have gained confidence in its use with others, you should have no problem committing yourself to using it as a learning strategy. The most traditional way to hypnotize yourself is to start by putting yourself in a comfortable position. It does not matter whether you are lying down or sitting up as long as you are comfortable. You need say nothing aloud, merely think your suggestions. Your eyes should be closed and relaxation enhanced if you take two or three deep breaths. Then think, Now I am going into the hypnotic state of consciousness. This is your first suggestion. Slowly repeat this suggestion in your mind three times, and you will begin to slip into hypnosis.

To achieve a slightly greater depth, simply say to yourself, I am going deeper, more and more relaxed. You may want to imagine yourself going down an escalator while you count backward from ten to zero, seeing yourself step down with each count. Picture yourself stepping off at the bottom when you reach zero and being ready to receive instructions.

The Spiegal Eye Roll is another induction that can be used effectively for self-hypnosis. This involves looking as high as possible with the eyes while at the same time taking a deep breath and closing the eyelids. After a moment, allow the eyes to lower while exhaling and visualizing a falling leaf. When the leaf finally falls to the ground, assume that you are in sufficient hypnosis to receive suggestions.

Although you should take for granted that you are entering hypnosis following these inductions (so as not to disrupt it with doubting or analytical thinking), it may be helpful to confirm the state with a simple suggestion for a finger levitation. After the induction, simply imagine a feeling of weightlessness in your index finger and see it lifting slightly upwards as though a helium balloon is tied to it. When you note the slight ideomotor movement, feel confident that you are ready for state-dependent learning.

Once this subtle change in consciousness occurs, begin giving yourself a single suggestion. The suggestion should have been previously determined, and it is best to learn one objective at a time. The suggestion may be in the form of a sentence or two, or it may be a visualized image of the desired result.

The specific goals for self-hypnosis preparation for personal medical emergencies may vary from person to person, depending on individual needs. One person may be especially negative reactive to the sight of their own blood. Another may lose control with the slightest feeling of pain. Still another may have problems when the emotion of guilt or anger is involved. Generally, however, everyone should program a reaction to a serious predicament that will allow for confident and automatic access to the following:

1. An immediate, objective appraisal of the situation and injuries (i.e., primary and secondary surveys)

2. A hopeful realization that the worst is over and that you have the capability of positively coping with the circumstances

3. The belief that you can and will give yourself hypnotic directives to control applicable involuntary nervous system functions so as to increase your chances for survival

THE SURVIVAL MIND-SET

Besides the specific objectives listed above, preparation for saving oneself during personal emergencies should include the development of a survival mind-set. This is the mind-set of those occasional victims at the scene of an emergency who seem to be in control no matter how badly they are hurt and regardless of the psychological intervention of the rescuer. Such a mind-set is valuable not only to survive personal injury or illness, but to persist when confronted with danger of any sort.

The following list gives six of the most important mind-set beliefs for optimal perseverance and personal growth in the face of danger. Look at each one, and see how your current belief compares to it. If they differ, imagine (or remember) the loss of control your belief could have (or had) in a specific survival situation. Do this until the inappropriateness of such a belief becomes obvious. Next, replace this view of reality with the one that is listed. Now, using self-hypnosis, visualize the gain in control that comes from the new assumption.

With this kind of mental practice, the new belief system will automatically help you maintain control the next time fear or circumstance calls for such action.

1. *When the emotion of fear comes forth, it is better to focus on the present task at hand than on either the past or the future.* "The point of power is in the present." If you believe this, you have an inexhaustible realm of ability at your command. When thoughts are focused on an immediate task, rather than on past events or imagined futures, you become unconsciously aware of many facets of your environment. If your thoughts are in the past or future, all you will have in the present is your fear. When fear comes, let it do no more than stimulate the adrenalin for your actions. Concentrate not on the fear, but on the immediate skills, work, and action. New, positive emotions will then follow the nature of your concentration, and your fear will disappear.

2. *Everything has a humorous side, and it is always worth looking for.* One of the positive emotions that can emerge when you concentrate in the present is laughter. A sense of humor has brought more people through difficult times than perhaps any other mental perspective. A humorous angle is embedded in all of life's predicaments. Being able to take yourself seriously and laugh at yourself at the same time is, at first, an elusive skill. But, with practice, a sense of humor will emerge spontaneously.

3. *Imagination is more powerful than determination.* Although you could walk along a 4-inch plank lying on the ground, you probably could not do this if it were suspended a hundred feet in the air, even if you were offered a great deal of money. Regardless of the knowledge that you have the ability and the determination to earn the money, your imagined possibility of falling would probably be the controlling factor. Survival is seldom a matter of willpower, but of imagination—to know what we ought to turn our wills toward.

4. *There are usually more than two alternatives.* There is a common mind-set in which an individual automatically assumes that there are

only two ways a situation can be resolved, and he limits himself to two ways of responding to a problem. This differs from the mind-set that understands there are usually several ways of reacting to a particular situation.

5. *Differentiation is as important as generalization.* Generalization is a learning strategy necessary for survival. But if your belief system does not also allow for differentiation, then optimal adaptation to stress is not likely to occur. Consider the following example.

Let us say you are lost and injured in a remote area. The land is hot and dry, and there have been wildland fire danger warnings posted. You smell smoke, and, using generalization alone, you now believe, on top of all your other troubles, you are going to be caught in a forest fire. So you run in the opposite direction, becoming further lost.

If your mind-set included differentiation, however, you would have considered the possibility that the smoke was from a large campfire, built by people who could have helped you. You would have looked for clues to determine the truth about the fire, and as a result, your life would have been saved.

6. *How we label things influences our reaction to them.* Labeling things is an important aspect of human communication, but during emergencies it can get us into trouble. When we label, we evaluate and predict, often erroneously. Most people are not aware of how much arbitrary labeling of situations—whether in the form of self-statements or with statements to others—can influence outcomes. With this new belief in mind, you can change problems into challenges, liabilities into assets, difficulties into opportunities, and a canteen that is half empty into one that is half full.

EMPOWERING OTHERS

Until you have spent many years practicing with self-hypnosis, it is easier to achieve profound results if you can empower someone else to give you hypnotic suggestions. We now know that the mind can manage the pain of a deep second-degree burn and can modify the inflammatory response in such a way as to significantly enhance healing. But it takes more confidence to give oneself the suggestions than to allow someone else to offer the appropriate suggestions.

Perhaps this is so because the left brain is less active when it is not responsible for structuring the correct directives, thus allowing a higher degree of receptivity from the right brain. Maybe it has to do with the phenomenon of rapport discussed in Chapter 3. Or perhaps it is because our earliest sense of protection came from the soothing words of those who took care of us. In any event, if it is possible to empower someone else at the emergency scene to use hypnosis to help you, do so. Of course, it is best if the other person has already been trained in using hypnosis, but if not, she can simply repeat the suggestions you propose.

GROUP SURVIVAL

Whether saving yourself from medical jeopardy or environmental risk at the emergency scene, the proper mind-set combined with the practiced ability to self-direct nervous system functions (or to instruct others to do so for you) can be a matter of life or death. Remember also that your ability to effectively use hypnosis with others may also help save your own life. In the following anecdote, note how one person's attitude and skills in this regard may have been responsible for saving an entire expedition.

Situation:

It was to be an adventure of a lifetime: six experienced river runners paddling an Avon inflatable raft down the uncharted Rio Ruique River through Mexico's Copper Canyon. Just reaching the water from the rim at El Divisidero was a challenge.

But when the rains started and the river began to rise, all six began to worry. And when the river turned a corner and disappeared into a drainage hole at the bottom of a large boulder, holding the raft fast at the entrance, the team began to pray. Each had enough experience to know they would never be able to get the boat away from the powerful force pulling it turbulently into the hole. Fortunately, they managed to climb the boulder to relative safety—all but the last person.

Just as Dan Brydon, the group leader, stepped on a pontoon to reach for a rock ledge, the boat surged and threw him into the hole. Down and under he went, disappearing for almost five seconds before popping up on the other side of the massive rock. As his friends grab him, they notice the dark red blood pulsing out of a small artery in his lip and can see that the angle of his shoulder is abnormal. Dan is barely conscious. As they lift him to the rock, a look of desperation begins to cover their faces.

Bill Hargrave's face is an exception. He has taken a first responder course that taught that all frightened emergency patients enter into a state of spontaneous hypnosis, making them hypersuggestible to confident directives. Bill positions himself next to Dan and speaks with authority and conviction:

Dan, listen to me! You just went through the hole and came up with some scratches and an injured shoulder. But the worst is over now! Go ahead and allow all your body systems to return to normal, and we'll get you out of here as best we can.

Dan opens his eyes, and, managing a courageous moment of humor, queries as to just how they are going to get off the rock and out of the 14,000-foot canyon. Then he winces in pain and almost chokes on the blood dripping into his throat.
  Bill continues with his matter-of-fact communication:

First things first, ol' buddy. I want to check you over to see how you're doing. Right now I want you to take a deep, relaxing breath. [Dan immediately responds.] Good. Now notice that relaxation beginning to flood through your body, keeping it warm and healthy. Now, when I count to three, I want you to go ahead and stop the bleeding in your lip. One, two, three.

Amazingly, the bleeding ceases. Bill dispassionately acknowledges Dan's success and continues with his survey. When he gets to the shoulder, he sees that it is dislocated. Bill speaks sincerely and with respect.

Dan, your shoulder is dislocated. If we are to get out of here, though, you'd be better off to have it back in place. Now, listen to me carefully. With your help, we can easily allow the joint to reconnect. All you need to do is relax the muscles around the shoulder.

Bill quietly orders several others to help position Dan and his arm. As they move him, he screams in pain. At that moment, Bill looks directly at Dan and says, "Dan, will you do what I say?"
  Dan's scream fades and the smoothness of his face returns. Bill begins gently touching the shoulder area and tells Dan to notice how relaxed and limp the whole area is becoming. He then directs him to maintain that feeling of looseness as they move his arm. With a minimum of effort, Bill pulls Dan's arm out and puts it back into place.
  After rigging a swatch and sling for Dan's arm and assuring him that he can walk, the group ponders their predicament. The water is rising rapidly, and the flow is approaching 10,000 cubic feet per second. Their only chance is to climb a precarious route from the rock to a trail that appears to head up the canyon. When Bill suggests that they had better start moving, he notices the look

of fear on his companion's faces. With the exception of Dan, they seem frozen to the rock.

Dan then speaks to the group, almost yelling so as to be heard above the roar of the rapids forming below them and the sound of rain rattling against their helmets. "I know we are all frightened, but we can all, even me, make it to the trail before the river gets much higher. I want you to watch me carefully and follow the exact path that I take." Dan then specifies the order in which the group is to proceed up the narrow route. When everyone safely reaches a well-worn jungle trail, he congratulates the team and directs an uneventful two-day trek to a small village near the top of the canyon.

QUESTION

List and describe five survival mind-set beliefs.

The empires of the future are the empires of the mind.
—Winston Churchill

Faith is a practical habit, which, like every other, is strengthened and increased by continual exercise, meditation, and prayer.
—Robert Hall

19 Saving the Planet

The underlying principle of language and thoughts that can dramatically influence the biology of people can also affect the ecology of our planet. This chapter shows how.

The human animal is a microcosm of the planet earth. We are made of the same mixtures of water and minerals. We both have great adaptability, yet our health depends upon a harmonious balance of many natural systems. Though we humans are slow to respond to emergencies that unfold in slow motion, we might agree that saving the planet is a worthwhile objective. If so, you will note with interest that many of the same strategies of communication for patients can also make a difference in reversing some of the destructive insults from which our planet is suffering. Sam Keen says this more poetically in his book, *The Passionate Life*, when he says, "The terrible and promising conclusion we must draw is that we will create a world that gives us evidence to support the metaphors by which we live."

It has been said that we are not suffering an energy crisis, but an intelligence crisis. Perhaps it would be more accurate to call it an imagery crisis. Just as negative images can negate survival mechanisms in the emergency patient, negative images can also create a self-fulfilling prophecy for the planet. Similarly, as positive images can create optimal survival conditions for the mind-body complex, they may be able to influence the health of the planet.

If the analogy about humans and the earth is not sufficiently convincing, or if you have difficulty comparing the influence of communication on the autonomic nervous system with its influence on such things as pollution, the depletion of natural resources, or war, consider the logic of physics.

THE NEW PHYSICS

The new physics reveals that energy is not constant, but comes in lumps and bumps called *quanta*. These *quantum* gaps and jumps in the energy continuum defy our ordinary perception of space and time. They connect actions, places, ideas, and moments in ways that no one has been able to explain adequately. In fact, these quantum are so intimately interrelated that the eminent physicist, Sir Arthur Addington, has said, "When the electron vibrates, the universe shakes."

But how does quantum mechanics support the hypothesis that image-producing communication can affect the health of the planet? Well, first of all, we must also note that the new physics says that consciousness is a form of energy. It too, then, is interrelated to all actions, places, ideas, and moments. Since by consciousness we are linked to everything, we also influence everything. Just as the atoms that comprise our cells are interrelated to the atoms that comprise all other structures, our thoughts are also interactive. The British physicist, Sir James Jeans, described it well as far back as in the 1940s:

Today there is a wide measurement of agreement . . . that the stream of knowledge is heading toward a nonmechanical reality; the universe begins to look more like a great thought than like a great machine. Mind no longer appears as an accidental intruder into the realm of matter; we are beginning to suspect that we ought rather to hail it as the creator and governor of the realm of matter.

Another way to understand the effect of your thoughts and images on the universe around you is to recall how your own negative mood can affect people with whom you come in contact. Similarly, remember how your good mood can have a positive effect. Note that your words and body language as well as your mood and thoughts triggered the reactions.

All of this is to say that each of us has a way, through our thoughts, images, and daily communication, to alter the course of events that shapes the world picture. Unfortunately, most of us have been expressing our communication in a negative way. How easy this is to do when so many horrible things are being communicated to us through the media. Reports of ozone layer disruption, the greenhouse effect, food, water, and air pollution, traffic problems and crime, energy crisis, and war, are heard or read almost daily. When we respond to these reports, however, we do not have to join in the negativity. We can reframe the problem and change the images that are being projected.

> *Situation:*
> *You have just returned from a hectic commute in traffic. When you arrive home you read in the newspaper that the number of automobiles in your area will double in two years. Then you hear on the radio that pollution from auto exhausts is most responsible for the depletion of the ozone layer. At this point you will probably make a negative comment about the future of the planet. In this situation, you are the rescuer.*

> Man, we're not going to be able to breathe the air outside our door in five years!

> *With this statement you are contributing to the self-fulfilling prophesy that many others are probably duplicating at the same moment. If, however, you reframe the problem as a challenge or an opportunity with a hopeful conclusion, as you have learned to do with your emergency patients, your contribution to the mass energy or consciousness can be positive:*

You know, the pollution from automobiles has been getting worse each year. We really need to do something to make the situation better. I read about an inventor who is trying to develop the capability to economically use helium as a fuel for cars so that the exhaust would be pure oxygen. Wouldn't it be neat if the air got better because of automobile exhaust instead of worse? We'll find an alternative, don't worry.

If our hypothesis, based on the facts regarding imagery, positive transference, quantum mechanics, the energy of consciousness, and the impact of language, has any merit at all, then this simple reframing, if done by enough people, can significantly create an environment in which new solutions to the pollution problem will be more likely.

In addition to rephrasing the bad news into an opportunity for positive change, there are other things that you can do to help assure that your images for the planet are optimal. Of course, there are also many actions you can take. For example, recycling, buying fuel-economical cars, conserving water, boycotting companies that are irresponsible, writing your congressman when appropriate, and so on—all are important. The positive images that you hold, however, when joined with those of others, may make the biggest difference in the long run.

GUIDELINES FOR POSITIVE IMAGES

Try your best to follow the guidelines and directives below along with the many others who are reading this book, and see what happens.

1. *Surround yourself with optimistic people.* Just as living cells have structure, react to stimuli, and organize according to their own classification, so do thoughts. Thoughts thrive on association. They magnetically attract others like themselves and repel those considered to be enemies. If you spend your time listening to the criticisms, complaints, and doomsday projections of people, soon you will be joining them in this kind of communication. Ask your friends to change the subject if they cannot say something positive, or leave the room until they do.

2. *Search for the hopeful viewpoint when you read or listen to radio or TV.* It may not be easy to find, but you will be surprised at how often you might have missed it in the past. More importantly, investigate

the origins of your negative beliefs. Remember that beliefs are the foundation of images. If your beliefs are based on old bias or propaganda, your images will tend to perpetuate the negative effect of these ideas.

3. *Pay attention to your self-talk.* You communicate hundreds of words to yourself, without selectivity, every few minutes. Some of these words reinforce negative emotions and beliefs about yourself and the world. Listen to yourself and change the negative self-statements to positive ones.

4. *Utilize the power of repetition.* It is no secret why most of us use the same words to complete the sentence, "Things go better with _____." You do not need a multimillion dollar budget, however, to repeat optimistic statements to yourself or others often enough for them to take hold of your imagination.

5. *Take time when you visualize to do something for the planet.* Most of us use such opportunities to manage our stress, enhance our performance, or prepare for a crisis. We tend to leave the fate of the planet out of our positive images. Once in a while, take a few minutes and use self-hypnosis-type mental processes to create a positive image for the world. Be general, or use your knowledge to focus on specific solutions.

In addition to the above, making a habit of the following basic qualities will promote the kinds of positive images that bring forth success. Embracing these qualities as you address the world picture will help assure that you are significantly contributing to the health of the planet.

6. *Practice optimism.* See the glass as half full instead of half empty. Turn problems into opportunities. Focus on the rewards of success rather than on the penalties of failure. Encourage and praise more often than you criticize. Help others realize that life on this planet is really worth saving.

7. *Laugh and sing more often.* Remember that laughter is universal. It connects people in an obvious way. It is also contagious. Laugh daily, even if you do not think there is anything to laugh about. Neither your body nor the people around you will know the difference, and all will benefit. Also, laughing is a catharsis. So when bad news strikes, it is a good way to rid yourself of it.

8. *Be aware.* Do not avoid bad news by hiding from it. Become educated about the alternatives for positive change so you can focus your images and communication. Remain open-minded. Trust your

intuition as you do your logic. Experience nature and risk adventure so that you truly feel a part of the universe.

9. *Emphasize love.* Treat all living creatures with kindness. Do not exploit others. Give your time and your energy to others, and remember to start with your inner circle of family and friends. Love yourself also, and love every moment as though it were your last.

10. *Remember to think in the present progressive tense.* By "becoming" in the now you remain in control. We have no control over the past or the future, only, to some measure, of the present. Although you can have images of a positive future, and you can review pleasant memories of the past, your mental concentration is the most effective when images are "becoming alive now."

11. *Cooperate with your fellows as best you can.* A sense of commitment to the planet is important if it is to survive. When survival and growth is no longer an issue, it is a temptation to focus on our own pursuit for pleasure. Our society must remember that it was cooperation that got it to the top. Develop mutual support systems when and wherever you can.

12. *Be positively motivated rather than negatively motivated.* Focus on the rewards of a healthy planet. Concentrate on solutions, not problems. If you fear an outcome, you subconsciously set that outcome up as a goal, and you will automatically strive toward it. Remember that we are motivated by our dominant thoughts. Since either fear or desire is behind most motivation, let desire be your green light for moving forward. Fear can be used to motivate people to stop doing something harmful to the planet, but only desire will provide the alternative.

13. *Do not give up.* Be persistent. Do not be disappointed if your positive attitude does not seem to change the world. All worthwhile efforts take time (perhaps a lifetime) and persistence.

14. *Be responsible.* We are individually responsible for how we respond to events and information. There is no benefit in just blaming others. If you think a corporation is doing something damaging to the environment, take some positive action. Each of us is accountable to life. We must decide on what values we attach to it, plan on ways to uphold those values, and set goals that actualize those values. Even if your goals are never fully realized, your continual pursuit of them makes you a role model for others to follow until the goal is ultimately accomplished.

Taking responsibility also means doing what you can to optimize your own physical health. Proper exercise and nutrition habits, avoidance of harmful substances, and so on show that you are a responsible person. How can you effectively complain about industrial pollution if you continue to pollute your own body?

It is sometimes difficult to accept responsibility when it seems like your single contribution is so relatively small. Remember, however, that you are part of a whole. When enough parts take responsibility, set goals, and pursue them with persistence, change will happen. It might take exactly one million people to turn the tide, but you could be that one-millionth individual!

Have confidence in the part you play in the scheme of things. Tap your dormant resources of power and use the tools of communication to stimulate that power in others. With that confidence and your sincere concern for all others, including the planet, positive things will happen. Whether you use thoughts and words to save an emergency patient, to treat a chronic disease, to inspire a child, or to reshape the planet, it is your choice to make.

QUESTION

How does the new physics support the use of positive words and images to influence the world situation?

Appendix 1

Countertransference

First responders and EMS personnel who utilize this book's approach to patient care will possibly risk *countertransference* more than those who continue to exclusively use a mechanistic, technical approach. Recognizing this possibility and taking appropriate remedial action will help prevent any lasting repercussions.

Countertransference refers to symptoms or stress passed on from patient to rescuer as a result of the shared involvement in the treatment efforts. When the first responder, EMT, or paramedic enters into the kind of rapport with a patient required to achieve the results that have been described, unconscious emotional contents can be transferred back and forth between the two individuals. This transference can touch unresolved or sensitive issues in the rescuer's unconscious that relate to fear of death, loss of relationships, parental control or abandonment, vulnerability, and so on. Occasionally, physical symptoms similar to those manifested by the patient can be temporarily exhibited by the rescuer.

The first step in preventing or removing countertransference hazards is to allow for full emotional involvement with the patient while still maintaining professional rapport. Do not allow any fears of countertransference or unconscious impulses to cause you to repress the unconscious field that you share with the patient.

The second step is to attempt to access and ventilate feelings and thoughts after the emergency incident is over. This can be done with friends or co-workers who have been trained to take this post-trauma exercise seriously.

The third step is to maintain a well-balanced lifestyle in general. Sufficient physical exercise to release physical tension and strengthen cardiovascular systems should be taken regularly. Alcohol usage should be limited and mind-altering drugs avoided entirely. Hobbies and interests unrelated to emergency rescue should also be developed.

And finally, countertransference should be viewed philosophically as an opportunity to realize that we all do indeed share in one another's thoughts and emotions to some degree. We all influence one another with our thoughts. With this understanding, learned over and over again from the countertransference phenomenon, we may better be able to perceive our connection with all things.

Appendix 2

Religious Considerations of Inner Mind Communication

During serious medical emergencies, religious beliefs are likely to come into the consciousness of the patient, the patient's family, or even the rescuer. In our American culture, where Christianity is the primary religion, it may be helpful to know that the teachings of Jesus support this book's assumption that words and thoughts can be healing.

For example, the major lesson in the Sermon on the Mount is that all experience is a manifestation of one's own conscious and subconscious mental states. In his interpretation of the Beatitudes, Emmet Fox states that Jesus's great law of the universe is just this—that what you think in your mind, you will produce in your experience. Scripture says it this way: "As within, so without."

Jesus also speaks of the "pure in heart." The word *heart* in the Bible usually means that part of humanity's mentality that modern psychology knows as the unconscious mind. Thus it is not enough to have conscious understanding that we can stop our bleeding. It is not until it is accepted by the unconscious mind, thus assimilated into the whole mentality, that it can actually be accomplished. As Jesus says, "As a man thinketh in his heart, so is he."

Jesus also teaches that fear and anger must be met at the unconscious level before healing can occur. "Let not your heart be troubled, neither let it be afraid." As long as there is fear or resentment, the emergency patient is not likely to manifest the objectives of your directives. So again we see that the strategies for calming and reassuring our patients at both the conscious and unconscious levels have support even in the Bible.

If you or your patients tend to grasp at Christian faith during medical emergencies, it is significant to note that Jesus calls human consciousness "the Secret Place." He says if we "think rightly" in this secret place, sooner or later all will be well on the outside. Shakespeare gives a similar message when he says, "There is nothing either good or bad but thinking makes it so." Whatever the rescuer or the patient gives his mental attention to will tend to manifest in some way. "If thine eye be single, thy whole body shall be full of light," is how Jesus phrased it.

Thus, in a very real way, the communication strategies that have been presented in this text might be considered to be grounded in the words of Jesus, as well as in the lessons of science and other great religious teachers. Since Christian ministers are often against approaches to healing that involve hypnotic language, remembering a few applicable lines of scripture might help displace this possible barrier to effective communication at a vital moment.

Bibliography

Cheek, David B., and Leslie LeCron. *Clinical Hypnotherapy*. New York: Grune & Stratton, 1968.

Chopra, Deepak. *Creating Health—Beyond Prevention, Toward Perfection*. Boston: Houghton Mifflin, 1987.

Chopra, Deepak. *Quantum Healing—Exploring the Frontiers of Mind/Body Medicine*. New York: Bantam, 1989.

Cousins, Norman. *Head First: The Biology of Hope*. New York: Dutton, 1990.

Dass, R., & P. Gorman. *How Can I Help? Stories and Reflections on Service*. New York: Knopf, 1987.

Esdaile, J. *Mesmerism in India*. Chicago: Psychic Research, 1902.

Green, Elmer, and Alyce Green. *Beyond Biofeedback*. New York: Delta, 1977.

Hay, Louise L. *You Can Heal Your Life*. Santa Monica: Hay House, 1984.

Oyle, Irving. *The Healing Mind*. Berkeley: Celestial Arts, 1979.

Peck, M. S. *The Road Less Traveled*. New York: Simon and Schuster, 1978.

Rossi, Ernie. *The Psycho-Biology of Mind/Body Healing*. New York: Norton, 1987.

Rossi, Ernie, & Cheek, David B. *Mind-Body Therapy*. New York: Norton, 1988.

Siegel, Bernie S. *Love, Medicine and Miracles*. New York: Harper & Row, 1986.

Index